Colitis

Understanding and Treating a Chronic Condition

Ethan D. Anderson

Xspurts.com

A New Zealand Designed Product

Other Versions Available

Why limit yourself to just one format?

This book is now available in physical, digital, and audiobook options.

Choose the way you love to read and dive into the story today. You won't regret it!

Digital ISBN: 9781776969777
Physical ISBN: 9781776969760
Audio ISBN:

To obtain a different format of this book at a discounted price, please get in touch with us at:

http://isbn.xspurts.com/

Contents

Have Questions / Comments? 1

Get Free Stuff 3

1. Introduction 5

2. What is Colitis? 7

3. The different types of Colitis 11

4. Ulcerative colitis 14

5. Crohn's disease 16

6. Chapter 6 18

7. Pseudomembranous colitis 20

8. Ischemic colitis 23

9. Microscopic colitis 26

10. Allergic colitis in infants 29

11. Who's at risk for colitis 32

12. How do you get Colitis 35

13. What are the symptoms of Colitis 37

14. What causes Colitis? 40

15. How can Colitis be prevented? 42

16. How is Colitis diagnosed? 44

17. How do you treat Colitis? 47

18. Alternative treatments for Colitis 52

19. What is the prognosis for Colitis 55

20. The role of diet in Colitis 58

21. The role of stress in Colitis 61

22. Exercise 65

23. What are the risks and complications associated with Colitis? 68

24. Living with Colitis 71

25. FAQ 83

Have Questions / Comments?

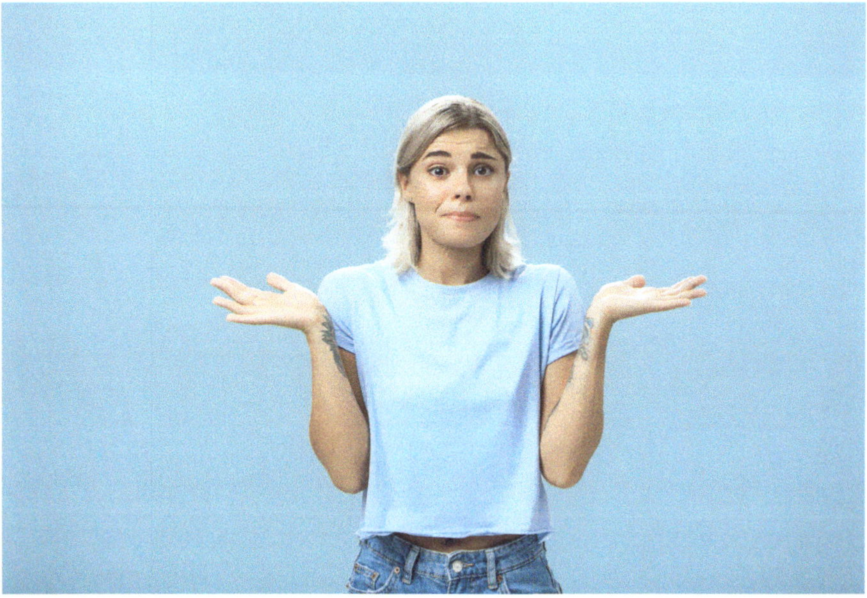

This book was designed to cover as much information as possible, but I know I have probably missed something, or some new amazing discovery has just come out.

If you notice something missing or have a question that I failed to answer, please get in touch and let me know. If I can, I will email you an answer and also update the book so others can also benefit from it.

Thanks For Being Awesome :)

Submit Your Questions / Comments At:

https://questions.xspurts.com

Get Free Stuff

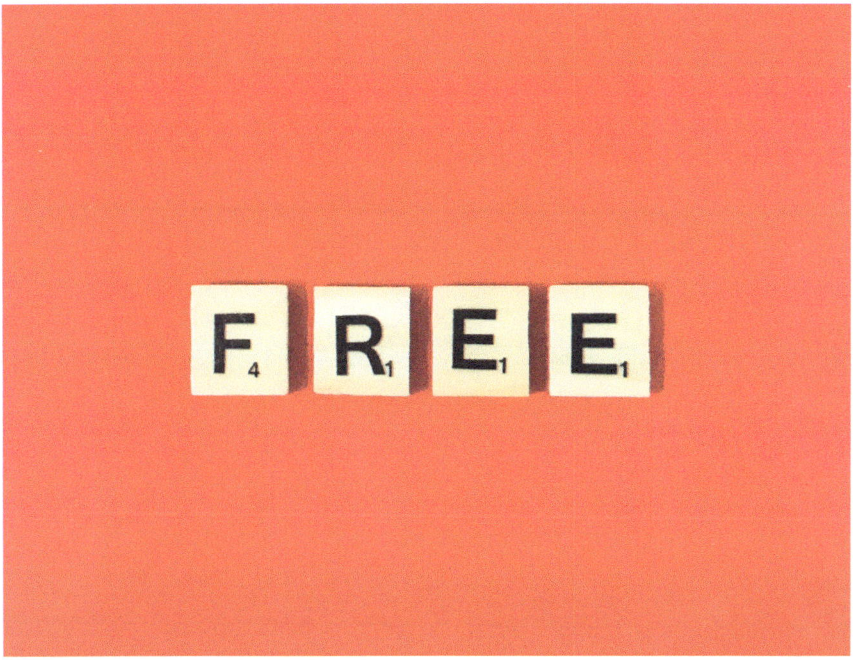

We love writing and have produced a huge number of books.

For being one of our amazing readers, we would love to offer you more books we have created, 100% free.

To claim this limited time special offer, simply go to the site below and enter your name and email address.

You will then receive loads (as we love our readers so much :) of our great books, content and audio direct to your email account, 100% free!

Get Loads of FREE Stuff at:

https://free.xspurts.com

Chapter One

Introduction

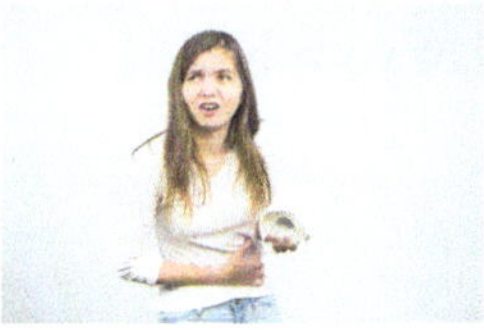

Colitis is a debilitating and painful condition that can drastically reduce the quality of life for those affected. This book aims to provide readers with everything they need to know about colitis, from preparing for diagnosis and treatment, to coping with the daily challenges of living with the condition.

Colitis is a chronic inflammatory condition that affects the colon, causing symptoms such as abdominal pain, diarrhea, and rectal bleeding. Living with colitis can be challenging, but with the right information and support, people with colitis can lead fulfilling lives.

In this book, "Colitis - Everything You Need To Know To Prepare For and Live with Colitis," we take a comprehensive look at this condition, covering everything from the causes and symptoms to diagnosis and treatment options.

Readers will learn about the different types of colitis, the symptoms and treatment options available, and how to manage the physical and emotional impact of the condition. With expert guidance and practical advice, this book will empower readers to take control of their health and wellbeing, and live their best life despite colitis.

Overall, this book is an essential guide for anyone living with colitis, as well as for family members and friends who want to understand and support loved ones with the condition. With the right information and support, people with colitis can lead fulfilling lives and navigate the challenges of this condition with confidence.

Whether you are newly diagnosed or have been living with colitis for some time, this book is a valuable resource that will help you understand your condition, manage your symptoms, and take control of your health.

Chapter Two

What is Colitis?

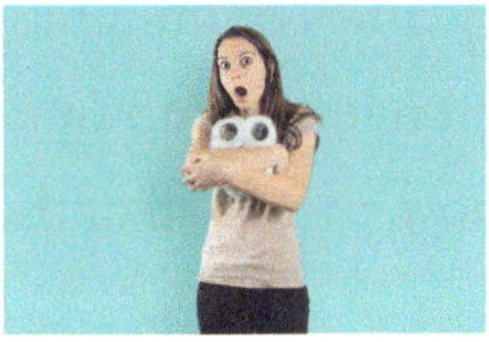

Colitis is a condition that affects the large intestine, also known as the colon. It is characterized by inflammation of the lining of the colon, which can cause a variety of symptoms including abdominal pain, diarrhea, and rectal bleeding.

There are several different types of colitis, each with their own specific causes and symptoms. The most common types include ulcerative colitis, Crohn's disease, and infectious colitis.

Ulcerative colitis is a chronic condition that causes inflammation and ulcers in the innermost lining of the colon. It typically affects the rectum and lower colon, but can also affect the entire colon. Symptoms of ulcerative colitis include abdominal pain, diarrhea, rectal bleeding, and weight loss.

Crohn's disease is a chronic condition that causes inflammation in the gastrointestinal tract, but most commonly affects the small intestine and colon. Crohn's disease can cause a variety of symptoms, including abdominal pain, diarrhea, rectal bleeding, weight loss, and fatigue.

Infectious colitis is caused by an infection in the colon, usually from bacteria such as E. coli or Salmonella. Symptoms include abdominal pain, diarrhea, and rectal bleeding. It usually clears up on its own within a few days or weeks, but can lead to more serious complications if left untreated.

Other types of colitis include ischemic colitis, which is caused by a lack of blood flow to the colon, and microscopic colitis, which is characterized by inflammation in the colon that can only be seen under a microscope.

Treatment for colitis depends on the type and severity of the condition. In some cases, medications such as anti-inflammatory drugs or immunosuppressants can be used to reduce inflammation and relieve symptoms. In more severe cases, surgery may be necessary to remove part or all of the affected colon.

It is important to note that colitis can lead to serious complications if left untreated, such as perforation of the colon, severe bleeding, and even cancer. If you suspect you may have colitis, it is important to see a doctor for a proper diagnosis and treatment plan.

Living with colitis can be challenging, but there are things you can do to manage your symptoms and improve your quality of life. Eating a healthy diet, staying hydrated, and getting regular exercise can all help to reduce inflammation and improve overall health. It's also important to work closely with your healthcare provider to develop a treatment plan that is right for you.

In conclusion, colitis is a condition that affects the large intestine and is characterized by inflammation of the lining of the colon. There are several different types of colitis, each with their own specific causes and symptoms. Treatment for colitis depends on the type and severity of the condition and it's important to see a doctor if you suspect you may have colitis. With the right treatment and lifestyle changes, people with colitis can lead fulfilling lives.

The Cause of Colitis

The exact cause of colitis is not fully understood, but research suggests that the disease is the result of an abnormal immune system response to the gut microbiome. The gut microbiome is the collection of microorganisms that reside in the digestive tract, including bacteria, viruses, and fungi. These microorganisms perform important functions in the body, such as aiding in digestion and nutrient absorption, and supporting the immune system.

In colitis, the immune system mistakenly identifies the gut microbiome as a threat and launches an attack against it, resulting in chronic inflammation and tissue damage. This immune response is thought to be triggered by a combination of genetic, environmental, and lifestyle factors.

Research has identified several genetic mutations that increase the risk of developing colitis, including variations in genes involved in immune system regulation and gut barrier function. Environmental factors such as diet, stress, and exposure to certain chemicals or toxins may also play a role in triggering the immune response in susceptible individuals.

In addition to the immune system's role in the development of colitis, there are several physiological factors that contribute to the disease. The lining of the colon and rectum is made up of several layers of cells, including the epithelial layer, which forms a barrier between the gut microbiome and the rest of the body. In colitis, this barrier becomes compromised, allowing bacteria and other harmful substances to penetrate the tissue and trigger an immune response.

The breakdown of the gut barrier can be caused by a variety of factors, including inflammation, oxidative stress, and pathogen invasion. Once the barrier is compromised, the immune system responds by sending immune cells to the site of the damage, where they release pro-inflammatory cytokines and other molecules that perpetuate the inflammatory response.

In addition to the breakdown of the gut barrier, there are several other physiological changes that occur in colitis. These include alterations in the gut microbiome, changes in the composition of mucus and other protective substances in the gut, and dysregulation of immune cell function.

Research has shown that the composition of the gut microbiome in individuals with colitis is different from that of healthy individuals. Specifically, there is a decrease in the diversity and abundance of beneficial bacteria, and an increase in harmful bacteria and other microorganisms. This dysbiosis can contribute to inflammation and tissue damage by altering the balance of pro- and anti-inflammatory molecules in the gut.

In addition to changes in the gut microbiome, individuals with colitis also experience changes in the composition and function of mucus and other protective substances in the gut. Mucus is a gel-like substance that lines the gut and helps protect it from harmful substances, including bacteria and other microorganisms. In colitis, the composition of mucus changes, making it less effective at protecting the gut and exacerbating inflammation.

Finally, dysregulation of immune cell function is another physiological factor that contributes to the development and progression of colitis. Immune cells in individuals with colitis are hyperactive and produce higher levels of pro-inflammatory cytokines and other molecules than in healthy individuals. This hyperactivity perpetuates the inflammatory response and contributes to tissue damage and other symptoms of the disease.

Chapter Three

The different types of Colitis

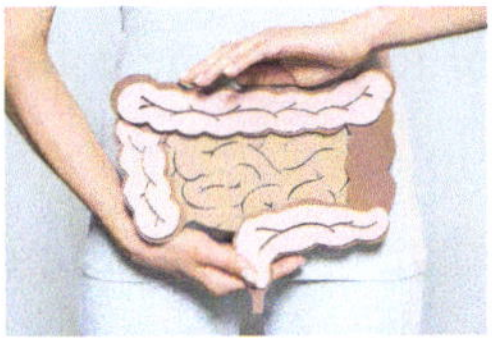

Colitis is a term used to describe inflammation of the colon. There are several different types of colitis, each with their own causes and symptoms. In this chapter, we'll take a closer look at the different types of colitis and what you should know about each one.

Ulcerative colitis: This is the most common type of colitis and is characterized by the presence of ulcers in the colon. The inflammation typically begins in the rectum and spreads upward. Symptoms of ulcerative colitis include diarrhea, abdominal pain, and rectal bleeding. Treatment for ulcerative colitis usually involves medications to reduce inflammation and to suppress the immune system.

Crohn's disease: This type of colitis is characterized by inflammation that can occur anywhere in the digestive tract, not just the colon. In addition to the symptoms of ulcerative colitis, Crohn's disease can also cause weight loss, fever, and fatigue. Treatment for Crohn's disease typically includes medications to reduce inflammation and to suppress the immune system. Surgery may also be needed in some cases.

Ischemic colitis: This type of colitis is caused by a lack of blood flow to the colon. It typically affects older adults and can be caused by things like blood clots or narrowed blood vessels. Symptoms of ischemic colitis include abdominal pain and diarrhea. Treatment for ischemic colitis typically involves restoring blood flow to the colon and managing any underlying conditions that may be contributing to the problem.

Microscopic colitis: This type of colitis is characterized by inflammation of the colon that cannot be seen with the naked eye. Instead, it can only be seen under a microscope. The two types of microscopic colitis are lymphocytic colitis and collagenous colitis. Symptoms of microscopic colitis include watery diarrhea, abdominal pain, and weight loss. Treatment typically involves medications to reduce inflammation and manage symptoms.

Infectious colitis: This type of colitis is caused by an infection in the colon. The most common cause is a bacterial infection, but viral and parasitic infections can also cause colitis. Symptoms of infectious colitis include diarrhea, abdominal cramping, and fever. Treatment for infectious colitis typically involves antibiotics or other medications to clear the infection.

Diverticulitis: This type of colitis is caused by small pockets or pouches that form in the lining of the colon. These pockets, called diverticula, can become inflamed and infected. Symptoms of diverticulitis include abdominal pain, fever, and constipation. Treatment for diverticulitis typically involves antibiotics and a diet that is low in fiber. Surgery may also be needed in some cases.

Collagenous colitis: This is a subtype of microscopic colitis and is characterized by thickening of the collagen layer in the colon. Symptoms of collagenous colitis include watery diarrhea, abdominal pain, and weight loss. Treatment typically involves medications to reduce inflammation and manage symptoms.

In conclusion, colitis is a term used to describe inflammation of the colon. There are several different types of colitis, each with their own causes and symptoms. If you suspect you may have colitis, it's important to see a doctor for an accurate diagnosis and appropriate treatment. Each type of colitis has its own unique set of symptoms, causes, and treatment options, and a doctor can help you understand your diagnosis and the best course of action for you.

Chapter Four

Ulcerative colitis

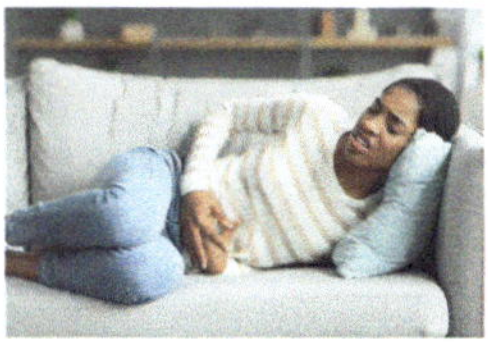

Ulcerative colitis is a type of inflammatory bowel disease (IBD) that affects the large intestine and rectum. It is characterized by inflammation, ulceration, and bleeding of the lining of the colon and rectum. The exact cause of ulcerative colitis is unknown, but it is thought to be a combination of genetic, environmental, and immune factors.

Symptoms of ulcerative colitis can vary from person to person, but common symptoms include diarrhea, abdominal pain and cramping, rectal bleeding, and weight loss. The severity of symptoms can also vary, with some people experiencing mild symptoms and others experiencing severe symptoms that can greatly impact their quality of life.

Diagnosis of ulcerative colitis typically begins with a physical examination and a review of the patient's medical history. Blood tests, stool tests, and imaging studies such as X-rays and colonoscopies may also be used to confirm the diagnosis.

Treatment for ulcerative colitis typically involves a combination of medications and lifestyle changes. Medications that are commonly used to treat ulcerative colitis include anti-inflammatory drugs, immune system suppressors, and biologic therapies. Lifestyle changes such as stress management and dietary adjustments can also be helpful in managing symptoms.

Surgery may be recommended for some patients with ulcerative colitis who do not respond to other treatments. The most common surgical procedure for ulcerative colitis is a colectomy, which involves removing the colon and rectum. This can provide relief from symptoms and prevent complications such as colon cancer.

It is important to note that while ulcerative colitis can be a chronic and potentially debilitating condition, with proper management and treatment, many people are able to lead normal and active lives.

Living with Ulcerative colitis can be challenging, but it is important to remember that you are not alone. Support groups and organizations can be a great resource for connecting with others who understand what you are going through. Additionally, working closely with your healthcare provider can help you develop a treatment plan that works for you and helps you manage your symptoms.

While there is no known cure for ulcerative colitis, with the right treatment plan and lifestyle changes, many people are able to live a normal and active life. It's important to work closely with your healthcare provider to develop a treatment plan that works for you and helps you manage your symptoms. Remember to take care of yourself, both physically and emotionally, and don't be afraid to reach out for support when you need it.

Chapter Five

Crohn's disease

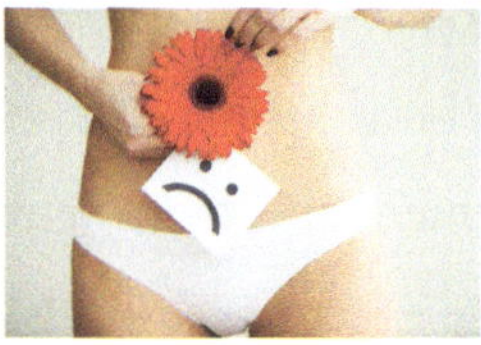

Crohn's disease is a chronic inflammatory bowel disease that can affect any part of the digestive tract from the mouth to the anus. The condition is characterized by inflammation and ulceration of the affected areas, which can cause a range of symptoms such as abdominal pain, diarrhea, rectal bleeding, weight loss, and fatigue.

The exact cause of Crohn's disease is not fully understood, but research suggests that it is the result of a combination of genetic, environmental, and immune system factors. Genetic mutations that affect the immune system's response to the gut microbiome are thought to increase the risk of developing Crohn's disease. Environmental factors such as diet, stress, and exposure to certain chemicals or toxins may also play a role in triggering the immune response in susceptible individuals.

The symptoms of Crohn's disease can vary depending on the location and severity of the inflammation. The most common symptoms include abdominal pain, diarrhea, rectal bleeding, weight loss, and fatigue. In severe cases, complications such as bowel obstruction, abscesses, and fistulas may occur.

There are several different types of Crohn's disease, based on the location of the inflammation. These include:

Chapter Six

- Ileocolitis: Inflammation in the ileum (the last part of the small intestine) and the colon.
- Ileitis: Inflammation in the ileum only.
- Gastroduodenal Crohn's disease: Inflammation in the stomach and duodenum (the first part of the small intestine).
- Jejunoileitis: Inflammation in the jejunum (the middle part of the small intestine) and the ileum.

Crohn's colitis: Inflammation in the colon only.

Treatment for Crohn's disease depends on the severity of the symptoms and the location and extent of the inflammation. The goals of treatment are to reduce inflammation, relieve symptoms, and prevent complications.

Medications are the most common treatment for Crohn's disease. These may include anti-inflammatory drugs such as corticosteroids or immunosuppressants, or biologic drugs that target specific molecules involved in the inflammatory response. In some cases, antibiotics may be prescribed to treat bacterial infections or other complications.

In addition to medications, dietary changes may be recommended to manage symptoms and prevent inflammation. Some people with Crohn's disease may benefit from a low-fiber or low-residue diet, while others may need to avoid certain foods that trigger symptoms.

In severe cases, surgery may be necessary to remove damaged or diseased portions of the digestive tract. Surgery is typically reserved for cases where medications and dietary changes have been ineffective at managing symptoms or preventing complications.

In conclusion, Crohn's disease is a chronic inflammatory bowel disease that can cause a range of symptoms and complications. The exact cause of the disease is not fully understood, but genetic, environmental, and immune system factors are thought to play a role. Treatment for Crohn's disease includes medications, dietary changes, and in some cases, surgery. With proper management, many people with Crohn's disease are able to live full and active lives.

Chapter Seven

Pseudomembranous colitis

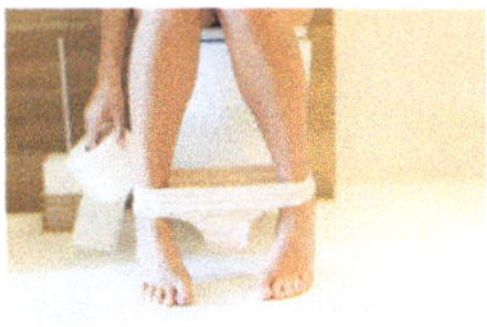

Pseudomembranous colitis, also known as antibiotic-associated colitis, is a condition that occurs when the healthy bacteria in your colon are destroyed by antibiotics, allowing harmful bacteria to overgrow and cause inflammation in the lining of the colon. This inflammation leads to the formation of a thick, creamy layer of pseudomembranes on the colon's surface, which is where the condition gets its name.

Symptoms of pseudomembranous colitis can include abdominal cramping and pain, diarrhea, fever, and dehydration. In severe cases, the condition can lead to life-threatening complications such as sepsis, toxic megacolon, and even colon perforation.

The most common cause of pseudomembranous colitis is the use of antibiotics. When you take antibiotics, they can kill not only the harmful bacteria that is making you sick, but also the beneficial bacteria that live in your gut. This can create an imbalance in the bacterial population of your colon, allowing harmful bacteria like Clostridium difficile (C. diff) to overgrow. C. diff is a type of bacteria that produces toxins that can cause inflammation and damage to the colon.

Another possible cause of pseudomembranous colitis is a weakened immune system. If your body's ability to fight off infection is compromised, you may be more susceptible to developing the condition. Other risk factors include advanced age, recent hospitalization or surgery, and the use of other medications that can affect the gut, such as nonsteroidal anti-inflammatory drugs (NSAIDs) or proton pump inhibitors (PPIs).

Diagnosis of pseudomembranous colitis typically involves a physical exam, a review of your medical history, and laboratory tests. Your doctor may perform a stool test to check for the presence of C. diff toxins, and may also order a colonoscopy or CT scan to get a better look at the inside of your colon.

Treatment for pseudomembranous colitis typically involves the use of antibiotics to kill the overgrowth of harmful bacteria. The most commonly used antibiotics for this condition are metronidazole and vancomycin. In some cases, your doctor may also recommend probiotics, which are beneficial bacteria that can help to restore the balance of your gut microbiome.

In addition to antibiotics and probiotics, your doctor may also recommend other treatments to help manage your symptoms and prevent complications. These may include fluid and electrolyte replacement to prevent dehydration, and anti-inflammatory medications to reduce inflammation in the colon.

While pseudomembranous colitis can be a serious condition, it is often treatable with antibiotics and other medications. However, it's important to take steps to prevent the condition from recurring, such as avoiding unnecessary antibiotic use and maintaining a healthy diet and lifestyle.

It's also worth noting that there's a link between taking antibiotics and developing pseudomembranous colitis, so it's important to have a conversation with your doctor about the risks and benefits of taking antibiotics.

If you're prescribed an antibiotic, be sure to take it exactly as directed, and don't hesitate to reach out to your doctor if you experience any unusual symptoms.

In conclusion, Pseudomembranous colitis is a serious condition that occurs when the healthy bacteria in your colon are destroyed by antibiotics, allowing harmful bacteria to overgrow and cause inflammation in the lining of the colon. The symptoms of the condition can include abdominal cramping and pain, diarrhea, fever, and dehydration, and in severe cases, it can lead to life-threatening complications such as sepsis, toxic megacolon, and even

Chapter Eight

Ischemic colitis

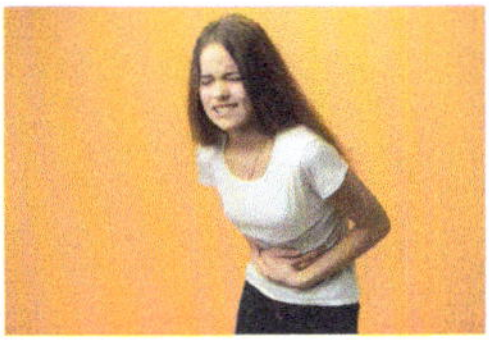

Ischemic colitis, also known as colon ischemia, is a medical condition that occurs when there is a lack of blood flow to the large intestine (colon). This lack of blood flow can lead to inflammation and damage of the colonic tissue, resulting in a wide range of symptoms that can range from mild to severe.

The most common cause of ischemic colitis is a blockage in the blood vessels that supply the colon. This blockage can be caused by a variety of factors, including arteriosclerosis (hardening of the arteries), blood clots, or other conditions that affect the blood vessels. In some cases, the blockage may be caused by an underlying medical condition, such as heart disease or diabetes.

Symptoms of ischemic colitis can include abdominal pain, diarrhea, and rectal bleeding. These symptoms can range from mild to severe and may come on suddenly or develop gradually over time. In some cases, the person may not experience any symptoms at all. However, if left untreated, ischemic colitis can lead to serious complications, such as perforation of the colon, which can be life-threatening.

Diagnosis of ischemic colitis typically begins with a physical examination and a review of the person's medical history. The healthcare provider may also order blood tests, stool tests, and imaging tests such as CT scan, colonoscopy, and angiography. These tests can help the healthcare provider to determine the cause of the ischemic colitis and to rule out other possible conditions that may be causing the symptoms.

Treatment for ischemic colitis depends on the underlying cause of the condition and the severity of the symptoms. In some cases, the person may be able to manage their symptoms with over-the-counter medications, such as anti-inflammatory drugs or antispasmodics. In more severe cases, the person may need to be hospitalized and may require surgery to remove the blockage or to repair any damage to the colon.

In addition to the treatment of ischemic colitis, the person should also focus on lifestyle changes that can help to improve blood flow and reduce the risk of complications. These changes may include quitting smoking, maintaining a healthy diet, and getting regular exercise.

Ischemic colitis can be a serious condition, but with proper treatment and management, most people are able to recover fully. If you have any symptoms of ischemic colitis, it is important to see a healthcare provider as soon as possible for diagnosis and treatment.

It's important to note that Ischemic colitis is usually more common in elderly population and people with underlying health conditions such as hypertension, heart disease, peripheral artery disease.It's also more common in people who are taking certain medications such as birth control pills, blood thinners, and nonsteroidal anti-inflammatory drugs (NSAIDs).

It's important to consult a doctor if you experience symptoms of Ischemic colitis, as it can be a serious condition if left untreated. Treatment will depend on the severity of the symptoms, but in most cases, it includes medications to reduce inflammation and pain, and in severe cases, surgery may be required.

Overall, Ischemic colitis is a condition that is caused by a lack of blood flow to the large intestine. It can cause a range of symptoms, and can lead to serious complications if left untreated. With proper diagnosis and treatment, however, most people are able to recover fully. If you have any symptoms of ischemic colitis, it is important to see a healthcare provider as soon as possible for diagnosis and treatment.

Chapter Nine

Microscopic colitis

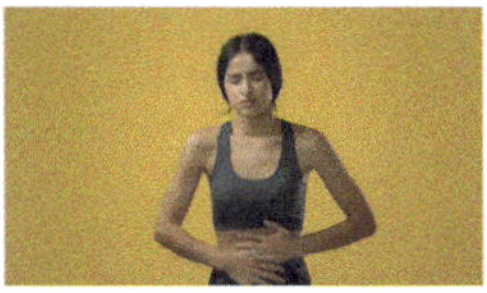

Microscopic colitis is a type of inflammatory bowel disease (IBD) that affects the large intestine, or colon. It's called "microscopic" because the inflammation can only be seen under a microscope, not with the naked eye. There are two types of microscopic colitis: collagenous colitis and lymphocytic colitis.

Collagenous colitis is characterized by a thickening of the layer of collagen under the lining of the colon. This thickening can cause inflammation and diarrhea. Lymphocytic colitis is characterized by an increase in the number of lymphocytes, a type of white blood cell, in the lining of the colon. This can also lead to inflammation and diarrhea.

Symptoms of microscopic colitis can include:

Chronic diarrhea (sometimes with as many as 20 bowel movements per day)

Abdominal pain and cramping

Bloating and gas

Fatigue

Weight loss

Many people with microscopic colitis also experience an urgent need to have a bowel movement, even if there is little or no stool to pass.

The exact cause of microscopic colitis is not known, but researchers believe that it may be triggered by a number of factors, including:

Certain medications (such as nonsteroidal anti-inflammatory drugs (NSAIDs)

Bacterial or viral infections

autoimmune diseases

Genetic factors

Hormonal changes

Diagnosis of microscopic colitis usually starts with a physical examination and a review of your medical history. Your doctor may also order a blood test, stool sample, or colonoscopy to rule out other conditions. A colonoscopy can help diagnose microscopic colitis by allowing your doctor to see the inside of your colon. A biopsy (removing a small sample of tissue) can also be taken during a colonoscopy and examined under a microscope to confirm the diagnosis.

Treatment for microscopic colitis typically includes:

Medications to reduce inflammation and diarrhea

Changing your diet (such as avoiding certain foods that can worsen diarrhea)

Fiber supplements to help regulate bowel movements

If you have microscopic colitis, it's important to work with your doctor to develop a treatment plan that's right for you. With the right treatment, most people with microscopic colitis are able to manage their symptoms and lead a normal life.

It's also important to note that microscopic colitis is a chronic condition, which means that symptoms may come and go. Even when symptoms are under control, it's important to continue working with your doctor to manage the condition. This may involve regular check-ups and adjustments to your treatment plan as needed.

In conclusion, Microscopic colitis is a type of inflammatory bowel disease (IBD) that affects the large intestine and is characterized by inflammation and diarrhea. There are two types of microscopic colitis: collagenous colitis and lymphocytic colitis. The exact cause of microscopic colitis is not known, but researchers believe that it may be triggered by a number of factors. Treatment for microscopic colitis typically includes medications to reduce inflammation and diarrhea, changing your diet and fiber supplements to help regulate bowel movements. It's important to work with your doctor to develop a treatment plan that's right for you and to continue managing the condition even when symptoms are under control.

Chapter Ten

Allergic colitis in infants

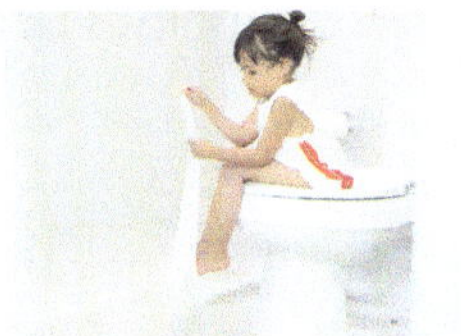

Allergic colitis in infants is a condition where an infant's large intestine becomes inflamed due to an allergic reaction to certain foods or other allergens. This can cause a variety of symptoms such as abdominal pain, diarrhea, and blood in the stool.

The exact cause of allergic colitis in infants is not well understood, but it is thought to be related to the immune system. In some cases, it may be caused by an allergic reaction to a specific food, such as cow's milk or soy. In other cases, it may be caused by a reaction to something in the environment, such as pet dander or dust mites.

Symptoms of allergic colitis in infants can vary depending on the severity of the condition. Some common symptoms include:

Abdominal pain or cramping

Diarrhea

Blood in the stool

Gas and bloating

Vomiting

Failure to thrive (in severe cases)

If you suspect that your infant has allergic colitis, it is important to seek medical attention right away. Your doctor will likely perform a physical examination and may order laboratory tests to help identify the cause of the inflammation. They may also order imaging tests such as an X-ray or an ultrasound to check for any structural abnormalities in the infant's large intestine.

Treatment for allergic colitis in infants will depend on the underlying cause of the condition. In some cases, your doctor may recommend eliminating certain foods from the infant's diet to see if that helps. This can be done by working with a nutritionist to create a special diet plan. For example, if cow's milk protein allergy is suspected, your doctor may recommend switching to a hypoallergenic formula or a soy-based formula.

If the cause of the allergic colitis is not food-related, your doctor may recommend medications to help reduce inflammation and relieve symptoms. Examples of these medications include steroids, such as prednisone, or anti-inflammatory drugs, such as mesalamine.

In some cases, infants with allergic colitis may also be prescribed a probiotic to help restore balance to the intestinal microbiome. Probiotics are beneficial bacteria that can help to improve the health of the gut and may help to reduce inflammation.

It is important to note that it may take some time to find the right treatment plan for your infant. Your doctor may need to make adjustments to the treatment plan as needed to find what works best for your child.

It's also important to note that, even with treatment, some infants may continue to experience symptoms of allergic colitis. In these cases, it is important to work closely with your doctor to manage the condition and to ensure that your child is getting the proper nutrition and care.

To prevent allergic colitis in infants, it is important to be aware of any potential food allergies or other allergies that your child may have. If you suspect that your child has a food allergy, it is important to work with a doctor to develop a special diet plan that eliminates the allergen. Additionally, if your child has other allergies, such as a dust mite allergy, it may be helpful to take steps to reduce exposure to the allergen.

In conclusion, Allergic colitis in infants is a condition where an infant's large intestine becomes inflamed due to an allergic reaction. It is a serious condition that can cause a variety of symptoms such as abdominal pain, diarrhea, and blood in the stool. If you suspect that your infant has allergic colitis, it is important to seek medical attention right away.

Chapter Eleven

Who's at risk for colitis

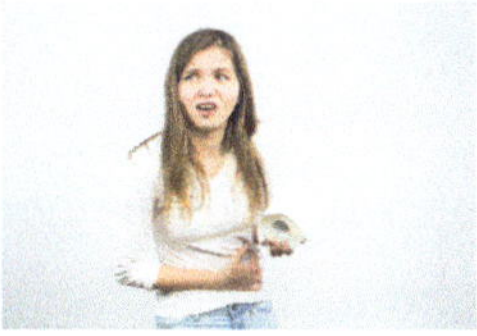

Colitis, also known as inflammatory bowel disease (IBD), is a condition that causes inflammation in the large intestine (colon) and/or the small intestine (small bowel). There are two main types of IBD: ulcerative colitis and Crohn's disease. Both types of IBD can cause similar symptoms, such as abdominal pain, diarrhea, and weight loss. However, the location and severity of the inflammation can differ between the two types.

While the exact cause of IBD is not fully understood, it is thought to be a combination of genetic, environmental, and immune system factors. Certain groups of people may be at a higher risk for developing colitis.

One group at risk for colitis are those with a family history of the condition. If a close relative (such as a parent, sibling, or child) has IBD, your risk of developing the condition is increased. Studies have shown that approximately 20-25% of people with IBD have a family member with the condition.

Another group at risk are those of certain ethnicities. Studies have shown that people of Jewish descent have a higher risk of developing IBD, particularly Crohn's disease. African Americans also have a slightly increased risk of developing ulcerative colitis.

Smoking is another risk factor for developing colitis. Studies have shown that smokers are more likely to develop Crohn's disease and that quitting smoking can reduce the risk of flare-ups in those who already have the condition.

Age also plays a role in the risk of developing colitis. IBD is most commonly diagnosed in people between the ages of 15 and 35, but it can occur at any age.

Certain medications are also associated with an increased risk of developing colitis. For example, people who take non-steroidal anti-inflammatory drugs (NSAIDs) such as ibuprofen or naproxen for a long period of time may be at a higher risk of developing the condition.

It's also important to note that people with certain underlying health conditions, such as autoimmune disorders or weakened immune systems, may be at a higher risk of developing colitis.

It's important to note that while certain groups of people may be at a higher risk for colitis, anyone can develop the condition. And if you have any symptoms of colitis, such as abdominal pain or blood in your stool, it's important to see a healthcare provider for proper diagnosis and treatment. While there is no cure for colitis, there are many effective treatments available to help manage the symptoms and reduce the risk of flare-ups. These include medications, dietary changes, and in some cases, surgery.

In conclusion, Colitis or IBD is an inflammatory condition that affects the large and small intestines. Though the exact cause of IBD is not fully understood, it is thought to be a combination of genetic, environmental, and immune system factors. Certain groups of people, such as those with a family history of the condition, certain ethnicities, smokers, certain age group, people on certain medications, and people with certain underlying health conditions are at a higher risk of developing colitis. But it's important to remember that anyone can develop the condition and if you have any symptoms of colitis, it's important to see a healthcare provider for proper diagnosis and treatment.

Chapter Twelve

How do you get Colitis

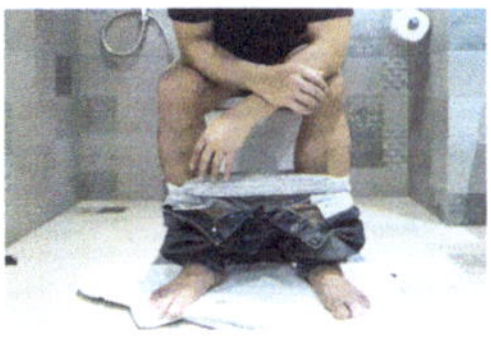

Colitis, also known as inflammatory bowel disease (IBD), is a condition that causes inflammation in the colon and rectum. While the exact cause of colitis is unknown, it is believed to be a combination of genetic, environmental, and immune factors.

One of the main risk factors for developing colitis is genetics. Studies have shown that people with a family history of IBD are more likely to develop the condition themselves. This suggests that there may be certain genetic factors that make individuals more susceptible to developing colitis.

Another risk factor for colitis is the environment. Research has shown that people living in urban areas or developed countries are more likely to develop IBD than those living in rural areas or developing countries. This suggests that certain environmental factors, such as diet, lifestyle, and pollution, may play a role in the development of colitis.

In addition, colitis is thought to be an immune-mediated disorder, which means that the immune system mistakenly attacks healthy cells in the colon and rectum, leading to inflammation and damage. Some researchers believe that certain microorganisms in the gut may trigger this immune response, leading to colitis.

Symptoms of colitis can include diarrhea, abdominal pain, cramping, and rectal bleeding. In severe cases, colitis can lead to weight loss, malnutrition, and anemia. If you suspect you have colitis, it is important to see a doctor for a proper diagnosis. Your doctor may perform a physical examination, blood tests, and imaging studies to rule out other conditions and make a definitive diagnosis.

Treatment for colitis typically involves a combination of medications, such as anti-inflammatory drugs, immunosuppressants, and antibiotics. In some cases, surgery may be necessary to remove the damaged portion of the colon.

Prevention of colitis is not well understood, but a healthy diet and lifestyle, such as regular exercise and stress management, may help to reduce the risk of developing the condition. Also, maintaining good hygiene and avoiding smoking are important to prevent the colitis.

In conclusion, colitis is a condition that causes inflammation in the colon and rectum and can be caused by a combination of genetic, environmental, and immune factors. If you suspect you have colitis, it is important to see a doctor for a proper diagnosis and treatment. While the cause of colitis is not fully understood, maintaining a healthy lifestyle may help to reduce the risk of developing the condition.

Chapter Thirteen

What are the symptoms of Colitis

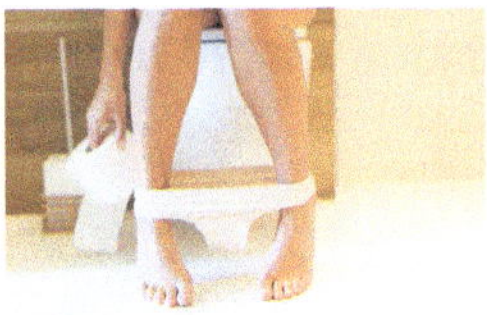

Colitis is a condition that affects the large intestine, also known as the colon. It is characterized by inflammation and irritation of the lining of the colon, which can lead to a variety of symptoms. Some of the most common symptoms of colitis include:

Diarrhea: This is one of the most common symptoms of colitis and can range from mild to severe. In some cases, the diarrhea may be bloody.

Abdominal pain: Many people with colitis experience abdominal pain, which can range from mild discomfort to severe cramping. This pain is usually located in the lower left side of the abdomen.

Fatigue: Colitis can cause fatigue due to the body's response to inflammation and the loss of fluids and nutrients.

Weight loss: Some people with colitis may experience weight loss due to the loss of appetite, malabsorption of nutrients, or diarrhea.

Rectal bleeding: Colitis can cause inflammation and ulceration of the lining of the rectum, which can lead to bleeding.

Anemia: Colitis can cause anemia due to the loss of blood from rectal bleeding.

Dehydration: Diarrhea and vomiting can cause dehydration, which can lead to symptoms such as dry mouth, dark urine, and dizziness.

Nausea and vomiting: Some people with colitis may experience nausea and vomiting, which can be caused by abdominal pain or dehydration.

Constipation: In some cases, colitis can cause constipation due to inflammation and narrowing of the colon.

-Fever: Some people with colitis may have fever as a result of the body's response to inflammation.

It's important to note that not everyone with colitis will experience all of these symptoms, and the severity of symptoms can vary from person to person. If you are experiencing any of these symptoms, it's important to see a doctor to rule out other conditions and to determine the best course of treatment.

Treatment for colitis typically involves the use of medications to reduce inflammation and to treat any complications that may arise. Some of the most commonly used medications for colitis include aminosalicylates, corticosteroids, and immunomodulators.

In some cases, surgery may be necessary to remove the affected portion of the colon or to create a diversion to allow the colon to heal. However, surgery is typically only considered when other treatments have been ineffective or when there is a risk of serious complications such as colon cancer.

It's important to work with your doctor to find the best treatment plan for you. This may involve making lifestyle changes such as eating a healthy diet, getting regular exercise, and managing stress.

If you have been diagnosed with colitis, it's also important to pay close attention to your body and to be aware of any changes in your symptoms. If you notice any changes or if your symptoms become more severe, be sure to contact your doctor right away. With the right treatment, many people with colitis are able to manage their symptoms and lead normal, healthy lives.

Chapter Fourteen

What causes Colitis?

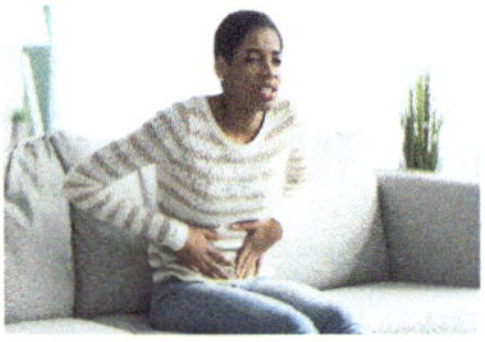

Colitis is a condition that affects the large intestine, also known as the colon. The colon's main function is to absorb water and electrolytes, and to store and eliminate waste. Colitis can be caused by a variety of factors, but the most common causes include infections, inflammatory conditions, and immune system disorders.

Infections: One of the most common causes of colitis is infection. Various types of bacteria, viruses, and parasites can infect the colon and cause inflammation. For example, the bacteria Clostridium difficile (C. difficile) is a common cause of colitis. This type of infection is usually caused by taking antibiotics, which can kill the good bacteria in the gut and allow C. difficile to overgrow. Other examples of infectious causes of colitis include Salmonella, Shigella, and Campylobacter.

Inflammatory conditions: Inflammatory conditions, such as ulcerative colitis and Crohn's disease, are also common causes of colitis. These are chronic conditions that cause inflammation in the gut, leading to symptoms such as diarrhea, abdominal pain, and weight loss. The exact cause of these inflammatory conditions is not known, but research suggests that a combination of genetic, environmental, and immune factors may play a role.

Immune system disorders: The immune system helps protect the body against infection and disease. In some cases, the immune system may mistakenly attack the body's own cells, leading to inflammation and damage. This can happen in the colon, leading to colitis. Examples of immune system disorders that can cause colitis include lupus and sarcoidosis.

Other causes: There are also other less common causes of colitis. For example, radiation therapy to the pelvic area can damage the colon and lead to colitis. Certain medications, such as nonsteroidal anti-inflammatory drugs (NSAIDs), can also cause colitis. Additionally, certain cancers, such as colon cancer, can cause symptoms similar to colitis.

In conclusion, Colitis can be caused by a variety of factors, including infections, inflammatory conditions, and immune system disorders. If you experience symptoms such as diarrhea, abdominal pain, and weight loss, it's important to see a doctor for a proper diagnosis and treatment. With the right treatment, most people with colitis can manage their symptoms and lead a normal life.

Chapter Fifteen

How can Colitis be prevented?

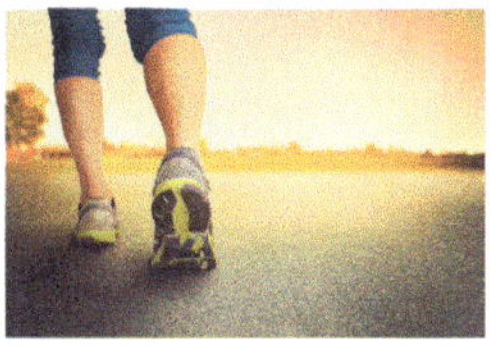

Colitis is an inflammation of the colon, which can cause a variety of symptoms including diarrhea, abdominal pain, and weight loss. While there is no surefire way to prevent colitis, there are several things you can do to lower your risk of developing the condition.

First and foremost, it's important to maintain a healthy diet. Eating a diet rich in fruits, vegetables, and whole grains can help keep your colon healthy and reduce your risk of colitis. It's also important to limit your intake of processed foods, sugary drinks, and red meat, as these have been linked to an increased risk of colitis.

Another way to lower your risk of colitis is to stay active and exercise regularly. Physical activity has been shown to improve gut health and reduce inflammation in the body. Aim for at least 30 minutes of moderate-intensity exercise, such as brisk walking or cycling, most days of the week.

Another important step in preventing colitis is to manage stress. Stress can trigger inflammation in the body and make existing colitis symptoms worse. There are many ways to manage stress, such as through meditation, yoga, deep breathing exercises, and therapy.

Additionally, it's important to pay attention to your symptoms and see your doctor if you notice any changes. If you have a family history of colitis or other inflammatory bowel diseases, you may want to talk to your doctor about getting screened for the condition.

If you are already suffering from colitis, your doctor may recommend certain medications to help manage your symptoms and reduce inflammation in the colon. These can include anti-inflammatory drugs, immunosuppressants, and biologic therapies.

In addition to these steps, there are also some natural remedies that may help prevent colitis. These include probiotics, which are beneficial bacteria that can help improve gut health, and omega-3 fatty acids, which have anti-inflammatory properties.

Overall, preventing colitis requires a multi-faceted approach that includes maintaining a healthy diet and exercise regimen, managing stress, and paying attention to your symptoms. If you are at risk for colitis or are already experiencing symptoms, talk to your doctor about the best ways to manage the condition and prevent it from getting worse.

It's important to note that the above information is for general prevention and management of colitis and should not be considered as a replacement for professional medical advice. It's always best to consult with a healthcare professional to determine the best course of treatment for you.

Chapter Sixteen

How is Colitis diagnosed?

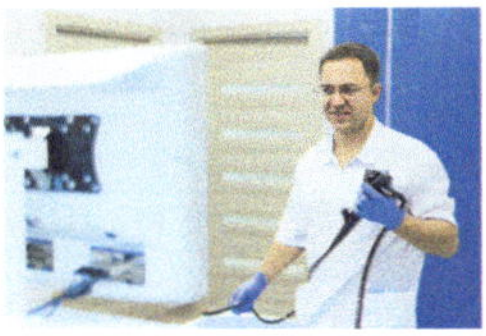

Colitis, which is inflammation of the colon, can be a tricky condition to diagnose. It's important to note that there are several different types of colitis, each with their own set of symptoms and diagnostic methods. However, in general, doctors will use a combination of physical exams, medical history, and various tests to diagnose colitis.

The first step in diagnosing colitis is typically a physical exam. During this exam, the doctor will check for signs of inflammation such as tenderness in the abdomen, changes in bowel movements, and blood in the stool. They may also use a stethoscope to listen to the sound of the intestines and check for any unusual noises.

Next, the doctor will ask about the patient's medical history. They'll want to know about any previous episodes of colitis or other inflammatory bowel diseases, as well as any family history of these conditions. They'll also ask about any other symptoms the patient may be experiencing, such as fatigue, weight loss, or anemia.

Once the physical exam and medical history have been completed, the doctor will likely order a series of tests to further investigate the patient's condition. These tests may include:

Blood tests: Blood tests can help check for anemia (low red blood cell count) or inflammation markers which may indicate the presence of colitis.

Stool tests: A stool test can check for blood, bacteria, or other abnormal substances in the stool that might indicate colitis or other intestinal problems.

Endoscopy: An endoscopy is a procedure where a thin, flexible tube with a camera on the end is inserted into the rectum and through the colon. This allows the doctor to see the inside of the colon and look for signs of inflammation or other abnormalities.

X-ray or CT scan: X-ray or CT scan can help the doctor to see if there is any thickening or narrowing of the colon that might indicate colitis.

Colonoscopy: A colonoscopy is similar to an endoscopy, but the doctor uses a longer tube to examine the entire colon. A colonoscopy can be used to detect ulcers, polyps, or other abnormal growths in the colon, as well as to take biopsies of suspicious areas for further testing.

It's worth noting that these are just a few of the many tests that may be used to diagnose colitis. The specific tests ordered will depend on the patient's symptoms, medical history, and other factors.

Once all of the test results are in, the doctor will be able to make a diagnosis of colitis. In some cases, the diagnosis may be clear-cut, but in other cases, it may be more difficult to determine the specific type of colitis the patient has. For example, Ulcerative Colitis and Crohn's disease are similar in many ways, but they have distinct differences.

In conclusion, diagnosing colitis can be a complex process that involves a combination of physical exams, medical history, and various tests. It's important to work closely with your doctor to determine the specific type of colitis you have and get the most appropriate treatment. With proper diagnosis, colitis can be treated and managed effectively, allowing you to live your life as normally as possible.

Chapter Seventeen

How do you treat Colitis?

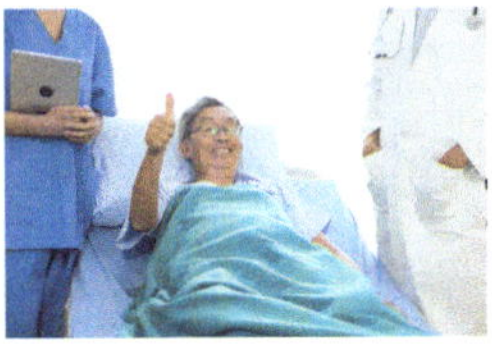

Treatment for colitis depends on the type and severity of the condition. But generally, the goal of treatment is to reduce inflammation, relieve symptoms, and prevent complications. Let's take a look at some of the most common treatment options for colitis.

Medications:

Anti-inflammatory drugs such as mesalamine and sulfasalazine are often used to reduce inflammation in the colon and relieve symptoms. Corticosteroids, such as prednisone, can also be used to reduce inflammation, but are usually only used for short-term treatment due to their potential side effects. Immunosuppressant drugs such as azathioprine and 6-mercaptopurine can also be used to reduce inflammation and prevent relapses.

Biological therapies:

Biological therapies such as infliximab and adalimumab are newer medications that are used to treat colitis. These drugs work by targeting specific proteins in the immune system that contribute to inflammation. They are typically used in people with moderate to severe colitis who have not responded to other treatments.

Surgery:

In some cases, surgery may be necessary to remove part or all of the affected colon. Surgery is usually recommended for people with severe colitis that has not responded to other treatments, or for people with complications such as a perforation or severe bleeding. Surgery can also be used to remove a portion of the colon that is affected by cancer.

Diet and lifestyle:

Eating a healthy diet, staying hydrated, and getting regular exercise can all help to reduce inflammation and improve overall health. Avoiding foods that can worsen symptoms, such as spicy or high-fiber foods, and consuming a diet rich in fruits, vegetables, and lean protein can help.

Probiotics:

Probiotics are live microorganisms that can provide health benefits when consumed in adequate amounts. Some studies have suggested that certain probiotics may be helpful in reducing symptoms of colitis. Probiotics may be used to help reduce inflammation and improve gut health.

Alternative therapies:

There are several alternative therapies that are sometimes used to treat colitis, including herbal supplements, acupuncture, and hypnotherapy. However, it is important to note that the effectiveness of these therapies has not been fully studied and more research is needed.

It is important to work closely with your healthcare provider to develop a treatment plan that is right for you. Treatment plans may need to be adjusted over time as symptoms change, and it is important to report any side effects or new symptoms to your healthcare provider.

Living with colitis can be challenging, but with the right treatment plan and lifestyle changes, people with colitis can lead fulfilling lives. It's also important to be aware of the signs and symptoms of colitis and to seek medical attention if they worsen, as colitis can lead to serious complications if left untreated.

In conclusion, treating colitis is a process and the treatment options are varied, it depends on the type and severity of the condition. Medications such as anti-inflammatory drugs, immunosuppressants, and biological therapies can help reduce inflammation and relieve symptoms. Surgery may be necessary in some cases, and diet and lifestyle changes, probiotics and alternative therapies can also play a role in managing the condition. It's important to work closely with your healthcare provider to develop a treatment plan that is right for you and to be aware of the signs and symptoms of colitis. With the right treatment and lifestyle changes, people with colitis can lead fulfilling lives.

Latest

Treaments

Options

There have been several recent advances in the treatment of colitis, including new medications and therapies that can help manage symptoms and prevent complications. Here are some of the latest treatment advances for colitis:

Biologic medications: Biologic medications are a type of medication that target specific molecules involved in the inflammatory response. These medications have revolutionized the treatment of colitis and other inflammatory bowel diseases, offering a more targeted and effective approach to managing symptoms. Some of the latest biologic medications for colitis include vedolizumab, ustekinumab, and tofacitinib.

Stem cell therapy: Stem cell therapy is a promising new treatment for colitis that involves using a patient's own stem cells to repair damaged tissue in the gut. The procedure involves collecting stem cells from the patient's bone marrow, processing them in a lab, and then injecting them into the damaged tissue in the gut. While still in the experimental stages, early results suggest that stem cell therapy may be a promising new approach to treating colitis.

Fecal microbiota transplantation (FMT): FMT is a procedure that involves transferring stool from a healthy donor into the gut of a patient with colitis. The goal of the procedure is to restore the balance of microorganisms in the gut and reduce inflammation. While still in the experimental stages, FMT has shown promise in managing symptoms and improving gut function in patients with colitis.

Diet and nutrition therapy: The role of diet and nutrition in the management of colitis is becoming increasingly recognized. Some studies suggest that certain diets, such as the low FODMAP diet or the specific carbohydrate diet, may help manage symptoms and reduce inflammation in patients with colitis. Additionally, some patients may benefit from nutritional supplements or specialized enteral nutrition formulas.

Telemedicine and remote monitoring: With the rise of telemedicine and remote monitoring technologies, patients with colitis now have more options for managing their condition from home. Remote monitoring devices can track symptoms, medication adherence, and other health metrics, allowing healthcare providers to make more informed treatment decisions and provide personalized care to patients.

Personalized medicine: With advances in genetic testing and precision medicine, there is increasing interest in developing personalized treatments for colitis. By analyzing a patient's genetic profile and other factors, healthcare providers may be able to tailor treatments to the individual, providing a more personalized and targeted approach to managing the condition.

Complementary and alternative therapies: While not a substitute for medical treatment, complementary and alternative therapies may be helpful in managing symptoms and improving overall well-being in patients with colitis. These may include acupuncture, massage therapy, yoga, and other mind-body approaches that have been shown to reduce stress and improve quality of life.

Wearable technology: Wearable technology such as smartwatches and fitness trackers can provide patients with colitis with valuable information about their health and activity levels. These devices can track symptoms, monitor heart rate and other vital signs, and provide reminders to take medications or engage in other self-care activities.

Patient education and support: As with any chronic condition, patient education and support are essential for managing colitis. Patients with colitis benefit from understanding their condition and treatment options, as well as having access to resources and support networks. Healthcare providers can play an important role in providing education and support to patients, as well as connecting them with patient advocacy groups and other resources.

Chapter Eighteen

Alternative treatments for Colitis

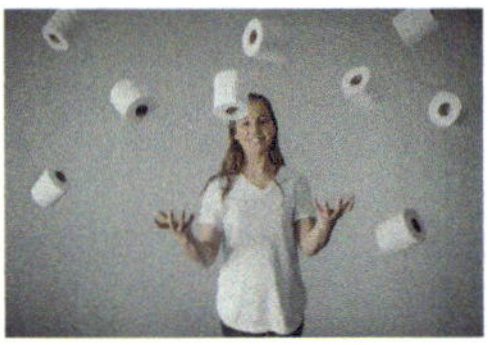

Colitis is a condition that causes inflammation in the colon and can be quite uncomfortable. While traditional medical treatments such as medication and surgery can be effective, many people also turn to alternative therapies to manage their symptoms and improve their overall health. In this chapter, we'll take a closer look at some of the most popular alternative treatments for colitis.

Diet and nutrition: What you eat can have a big impact on your colitis symptoms. Some people find that certain foods, such as processed foods, dairy products, and high-fiber foods, can trigger symptoms. Others find that a diet that is high in fruits, vegetables, and lean protein can help reduce inflammation and improve symptoms. If you're not sure what diet is best for you, consider working with a registered dietitian or a holistic nutritionist who can help you create a meal plan that works for you.

Probiotics: Probiotics are good bacteria that live in your gut and help keep your digestive system healthy. Some research suggests that taking probiotics can help reduce inflammation and improve symptoms of colitis. Probiotics can be found in fermented foods like yogurt, kefir, and sauerkraut, or they can be taken in supplement form.

Herbal supplements: There are a number of herbal supplements that are thought to have anti-inflammatory properties and may help reduce symptoms of colitis. Some of the most popular supplements include turmeric, which contains the anti-inflammatory compound curcumin, and boswellia, which is thought to reduce inflammation in the gut. It's always best to check with your healthcare provider before taking any supplement as some can interact with medication or have side effects.

Yoga and meditation: Yoga and meditation can be effective in reducing stress and tension, which can exacerbate colitis symptoms. Yoga can also help improve your overall health and well-being. Many people find that a regular yoga practice can help reduce symptoms and improve their quality of life.

Acupuncture: Acupuncture is a traditional Chinese medicine practice that involves the insertion of thin needles into specific points on the body. Some research suggests that acupuncture can help reduce inflammation and improve symptoms of colitis. However, it's important to find a qualified practitioner who has experience treating colitis.

Massage therapy: Massage therapy can help reduce muscle tension, which can be a contributing factor to colitis symptoms. It can also help to improve circulation and reduce inflammation. If you're interested in trying massage therapy, make sure to find a qualified therapist who has experience treating colitis.

Mind-body therapies: Mind-body therapies such as cognitive-behavioral therapy (CBT) and hypnotherapy can help you to manage stress and reduce symptoms of colitis. CBT can help you to change negative thoughts and behaviors that may be exacerbating your symptoms. Hypnotherapy can help you to relax and reduce stress, which can help to improve symptoms.

It's important to note that alternative treatments should not replace traditional medical treatments, but rather be used in addition to it. It's always best to consult with your healthcare provider before trying any new treatment, as some alternative treatments may interact with your medications or have potential side effects.

In conclusion, colitis is a condition that can be quite uncomfortable, and there are many alternative treatments that can help to reduce symptoms and improve overall health. Some of the most popular alternative treatments include diet and nutrition, probiotics, herbal supplements, yoga and meditation, acupuncture, massage therapy, and mind-body therapies. It's always best to consult with your healthcare provider before trying any new treatment, as some alternative treatments may interact with your medications or have potential side effects.

Chapter Nineteen

What is the prognosis for Colitis

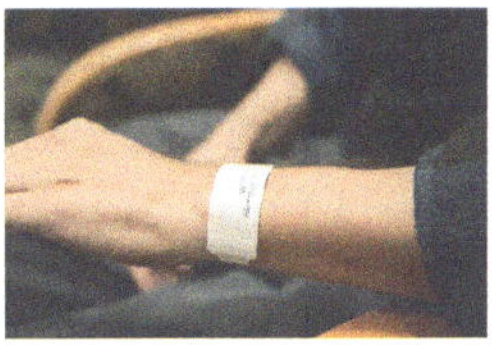

Ulcerative colitis, like other forms of inflammatory bowel disease (IBD), can be a chronic and unpredictable condition. The prognosis for colitis varies from person to person, depending on factors such as the severity of the disease, the patient's overall health, and how well the disease is managed.

In general, the prognosis for colitis is considered to be good, with many people achieving remission of symptoms with proper treatment and management. However, the disease may also have periods of flare-ups, where symptoms worsen and require more intensive treatment.

For some people, the disease may be more aggressive and difficult to control, leading to more frequent hospitalizations and an increased risk of complications such as colon cancer. In these cases, the prognosis may be less favorable.

One of the most important things you can do to improve your prognosis is to work closely with your healthcare provider to develop an effective treatment plan. This may involve a combination of medications, such as anti-inflammatory drugs, immune system suppressors, and biologic therapies. Lifestyle changes, such as stress management, dietary adjustments, and exercise, can also be helpful in managing symptoms.

Surgery may be recommended for some patients with colitis who do not respond to other treatments. The most common surgical procedure for ulcerative colitis is a colectomy, which involves removing the colon and rectum. This can provide relief from symptoms and prevent complications such as colon cancer.

It's important to note that even with treatment, some people may continue to experience symptoms and may need to make lifestyle adjustments to manage the disease. For example, some people may need to avoid certain foods, limit their alcohol and caffeine intake, or take steps to manage stress.

It's also important to be aware of the possible complications of colitis. Some of the most common complications include malnutrition, anemia, and osteoporosis, which can be caused by chronic inflammation, malabsorption and medication side effects.

Despite the challenges of living with colitis, it's important to remember that many people are able to lead normal and active lives with the disease. Support groups and organizations can be a great resource for connecting with others who understand what you're going through. Additionally, working closely with your healthcare provider can help you develop a treatment plan that works for you and helps you manage your symptoms.

It's important to remember that colitis is a chronic condition, and the prognosis can be different for each individual. With the right treatment plan, lifestyle changes, and support, many people are able to manage their symptoms and lead normal, active lives. However, it's also important to be aware that the disease may have periods of flare-ups, and that complications can occur. It's important to work closely with your healthcare provider to monitor your condition, and be aware of any changes or new symptoms that may occur.

In general, people with colitis, have a better quality of life with proper management of the disease, which includes taking medications as prescribed, following a healthy diet and exercise, and managing stress. With the right treatment plan and support, people with colitis can lead fulfilling lives and enjoy the things that matter most to them.

Chapter Twenty

The role of diet in Colitis

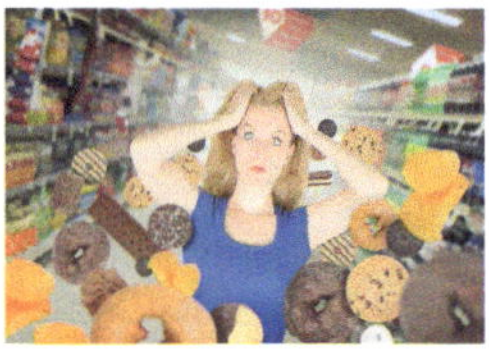

Diet plays a crucial role in managing colitis, a type of inflammatory bowel disease (IBD) that affects the colon. While there's no one-size-fits-all diet for colitis, certain foods and nutrients can help to reduce inflammation and alleviate symptoms.

One of the key dietary recommendations for colitis is to focus on anti-inflammatory foods. These include fruits, vegetables, whole grains, lean proteins, and healthy fats. Fruits and vegetables are particularly important, as they're rich in antioxidants and other nutrients that can help to reduce inflammation. Berries, leafy greens, and colorful produce like bell peppers and tomatoes are all great choices.

Whole grains, such as quinoa, brown rice, and oats, are also beneficial for colitis. They're rich in fiber and other nutrients that can help to promote healthy digestion and reduce inflammation.

Proteins are also an important part of the diet for colitis. Fish and seafood, in particular, are good sources of omega-3 fatty acids, which have anti-inflammatory properties. Other good sources of protein include lean meats, poultry, and plant-based options like beans and lentils.

Healthy fats, such as those found in avocados, nuts, and seeds, can also help to reduce inflammation and improve symptoms of colitis.

Another important aspect of diet for colitis is to be mindful of portion sizes. Eating smaller, more frequent meals throughout the day can help to prevent flare-ups and alleviate symptoms. Avoiding large, heavy meals can also help to reduce the stress on your digestive system.

Certain foods and beverages should be avoided or limited when managing colitis. These include processed foods, fried foods, high-fat meats, and sugary drinks. These types of foods can increase inflammation, exacerbate symptoms, and make it more difficult to manage the condition.

Caffeine and alcohol should also be avoided or limited, as they can irritate the gut and exacerbate symptoms of colitis.

It's also important to stay well-hydrated when managing colitis. Drinking plenty of water can help to keep the colon hydrated and reduce the risk of constipation and other digestive problems.

One of the most important things to keep in mind when managing colitis is that everyone's body is different and what works for one person may not work for another. It's important to work with a healthcare professional to come up with a diet plan that works for you. Additionally, it's important to note that some people with colitis may have food allergies or sensitivities, so it's important to pay attention to how different foods affect you.

A specific diet for colitis is the Specific Carbohydrate Diet (SCD) which eliminates certain carbohydrates and sugar, and focus on nutrient-dense whole foods to help reduce inflammation and promote healing in the gut. This diet eliminates grains, starchy vegetables, and processed foods and sugars, and allows only specific types of carbohydrates, such as those found in non-starchy vegetables and certain fruits.

Another specific diet is the Low FODMAP diet, which is used to manage symptoms of IBD, including colitis. FODMAP stands for fermentable oligosaccharides, disaccharides, monosaccharides, and polyols, which are types of carbohydrates that can be difficult to digest. The diet eliminates high-FODMAP foods, such as certain fruits, vegetables, grains, and dairy products, to reduce symptoms like gas, bloating, and diarrhea.

In conclusion, diet plays a crucial role in managing colitis, a type of inflammatory bowel disease (IBD) that affects the colon.

Chapter Twenty-One

The role of stress in Colitis

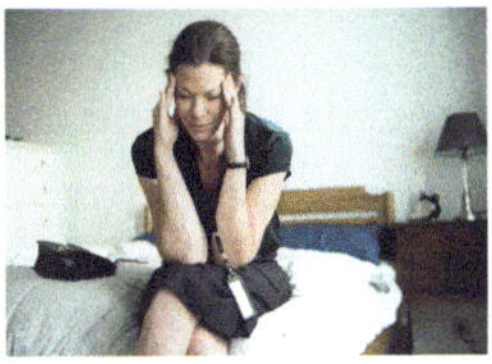

Colitis is an inflammatory condition that affects the large intestine, and it can cause a wide range of symptoms, including abdominal pain, diarrhea, and rectal bleeding. While the exact cause of colitis is not known, there is evidence that stress may play a role in the development and progression of the condition.

Stress is a normal part of life, but when it becomes chronic, it can take a toll on our physical and mental health. Stress can affect the immune system, making us more susceptible to infections and other health problems. It can also affect the gut, leading to changes in the gut microbiome and increased inflammation.

Research has shown that people with colitis are more likely to experience stress, and that stress can make their symptoms worse. In fact, studies have found that people with colitis have higher levels of the stress hormone cortisol in their blood, and that stress can cause flare-ups of colitis symptoms.

One way that stress may affect colitis is by altering the gut microbiome. The gut microbiome is the collection of microorganisms that live in the gut, and it plays a crucial role in maintaining our overall health. When we are stressed, the balance of the gut microbiome can become disrupted, leading to an overgrowth of harmful bacteria and increased inflammation. This can make colitis symptoms worse.

Another way that stress may affect colitis is by affecting the immune system. When we are stressed, our bodies release chemicals called inflammatory cytokines that can cause inflammation throughout the body. In people with colitis, this increased inflammation can lead to flare-ups of symptoms.

Stress can also affect the gut barrier, which is a layer of cells that line the gut and help to keep harmful substances from entering the body. When we are stressed, the gut barrier can become more permeable, which allows harmful substances to enter the body and contribute to inflammation and symptoms of colitis.

While stress can have a negative impact on colitis, it is important to note that stress is not the only cause of the condition. Colitis is a complex condition with multiple causes, including genetics, environmental factors, and gut microbiome.

Managing stress is an important part of treating and preventing colitis symptoms. There are a variety of different stress management techniques that can help, such as deep breathing exercises, meditation, and yoga.

Cognitive-behavioral therapy (CBT) is a form of psychotherapy that can help people to identify and change negative thought patterns and behaviors. CBT can help people to better cope with stress and reduce the risk of flare-ups of colitis symptoms.

Exercise is also a great way to manage stress and improve overall health. Regular exercise can help to reduce inflammation, improve gut health, and boost the immune system.

Diet also plays an important role in managing stress and colitis symptoms. A diet high in fiber and low in processed foods can help to support gut health and reduce inflammation.

In summary, stress plays a role in colitis, a condition that affects the large intestine and causes a wide range of symptoms. Stress can affect the gut microbiome, immune system, and gut barrier, leading to increased inflammation and symptoms flare-ups. While stress is not the only cause of colitis, managing stress is an important part of treating and preventing colitis symptoms. There are various techniques that can help to manage stress such as deep breathing exercises, meditation, yoga, and therapy. A healthy diet and regular exercise can also help to support gut health and reduce inflammation.

The Emotional Toll

Living with colitis can be challenging both physically and emotionally. The unpredictable nature of the disease can cause frustration, anxiety, and other negative emotions. However, it is possible to overcome these emotions and become stronger with time and effort.

One of the most important things to do when living with colitis is to seek support from friends, family, and healthcare professionals. Having a support system can help you feel less isolated and more understood. It is also important to educate yourself about the disease and its management strategies, such as medication, diet, and stress reduction techniques.

Another helpful strategy is to practice mindfulness and self-compassion. Mindfulness involves being present in the moment and accepting your thoughts and feelings without judgment. Self-compassion involves treating yourself with kindness and understanding, and recognizing that living with colitis is not your fault.

It is also important to maintain a healthy lifestyle, including regular exercise, healthy eating habits, and good sleep hygiene. These habits can help reduce stress, improve digestion, and boost overall well-being.

It is important to remember that everyone's experience with colitis is unique, and what works for one person may not work for another. Therefore, it is essential to work with your healthcare team to develop a personalized treatment plan that meets your specific needs.

It is also crucial to stay positive and hopeful, even when living with colitis can be challenging. While there is no cure for the disease, there are many effective treatments available that can help manage symptoms and improve quality of life.

In addition to medical treatments, it can be helpful to explore complementary therapies such as acupuncture, massage, and meditation. These therapies can help reduce stress and promote relaxation, which can have a positive impact on overall health and well-being.

Finally, it is important to remember that living with colitis can make you stronger and more resilient. By facing the challenges of the disease, you can develop a deeper sense of empathy, compassion, and gratitude. You can also learn to appreciate the small joys in life and find meaning in the face of adversity.

Living with colitis can be a daunting prospect, but it is important to remember that you are not alone. By seeking support, practicing self-care, and staying positive, you can overcome negative emotions and become stronger in the face of adversity. With the right approach, it is possible to live a fulfilling and meaningful life despite the challenges of the disease.

Chapter Twenty-Two

Exercise

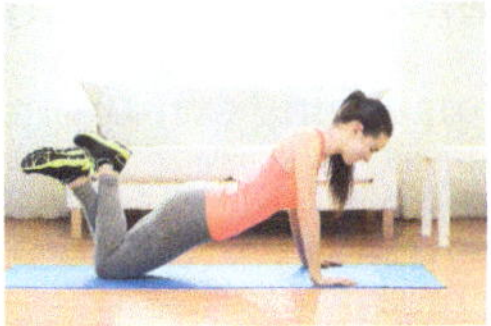

Exercise can be a valuable component of the treatment plan for colitis, as it can help manage symptoms, improve overall health, and reduce stress. Here are some ways that exercise can be used to treat colitis:

Reducing inflammation: Exercise has been shown to reduce inflammation throughout the body, including in the gut. By reducing inflammation, exercise may help manage symptoms in patients with colitis.

Improving gut function: Exercise can improve gut function by increasing blood flow to the digestive tract and promoting the movement of food through the intestines. This can help reduce symptoms such as constipation and diarrhea.

Boosting immune function: Regular exercise has been shown to boost immune function, which may be beneficial for patients with colitis who have an overactive immune system. By improving immune function, exercise may help reduce inflammation and prevent complications.

Reducing stress: Stress can exacerbate symptoms of colitis, so finding ways to reduce stress is an important part of managing the condition. Exercise is a great way to reduce stress and promote relaxation, which may help improve overall well-being in patients with colitis.

Improving mood: Exercise can also improve mood and reduce symptoms of anxiety and depression, which are common among patients with chronic conditions like colitis. By improving mood and reducing stress, exercise may help patients manage their condition more effectively.

Maintaining a healthy weight: Exercise can help individuals with colitis maintain a healthy weight, which is important for managing symptoms and preventing complications. Obesity has been linked to an increased risk of developing colitis and other inflammatory bowel diseases, so maintaining a healthy weight through exercise and diet may help reduce this risk.

Improving cardiovascular health: Exercise can improve cardiovascular health by strengthening the heart and improving circulation. This can be especially important for patients with colitis, as they may be at higher risk for cardiovascular disease due to chronic inflammation and other factors.

Enhancing quality of life: Exercise can enhance quality of life for patients with colitis by improving physical function, reducing symptoms, and promoting overall well-being. This can help patients maintain their independence and engage in activities they enjoy, which can be especially important for individuals with a chronic condition.

It's important to note that the type and intensity of exercise will vary depending on the individual and their symptoms. Some patients with colitis may benefit from low-intensity exercise such as walking or yoga, while others may be able to tolerate more high-intensity exercise such as running or weightlifting. It's important to work with a healthcare provider or a qualified exercise professional to develop an exercise plan that is safe and effective for the individual.

In conclusion, exercise can be a valuable part of the treatment plan for colitis. By reducing inflammation, improving gut function, boosting immune function, reducing stress, and improving mood, exercise may help manage symptoms and improve overall well-being in patients with colitis. As with any treatment approach, it's important to work with a healthcare provider to develop a safe and effective exercise plan that is tailored to the individual's needs and symptoms.

Chapter Twenty-Three

What are the risks and complications associated with Colitis?

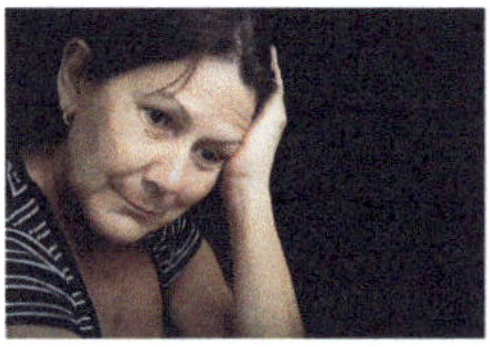

Colitis, also known as inflammatory bowel disease (IBD), is a chronic condition that causes inflammation in the lining of the colon and rectum. There are two main types of colitis: ulcerative colitis and Crohn's disease. While the causes of colitis are not entirely understood, it is believed to be a combination of genetic, environmental, and immune factors.

One of the most common risks associated with colitis is the development of ulcers in the colon and rectum. These ulcers can cause bleeding, pain, and diarrhea. In some cases, the ulcers can become infected, leading to a condition called colitis-associated sepsis. This can be life-threatening and requires immediate medical attention.

Another risk associated with colitis is the development of cancer of the colon and rectum. People with colitis have a higher risk of developing colon cancer because of the chronic inflammation in the colon. This risk is even higher for those who have had colitis for a long time or who have a family history of colon cancer. Regular colonoscopies and other screening tests can help detect colon cancer early, when it is most treatable.

Colitis can also cause other complications such as malnutrition, weight loss, and anemia. The chronic diarrhea and abdominal pain caused by colitis can make it difficult for people to eat and absorb nutrients properly. This can lead to malnutrition and weight loss. Anemia, a condition in which the body doesn't have enough red blood cells, can also develop due to blood loss from the ulcers.

Colitis can also affect other organs in the body, causing extra-intestinal manifestations. This can include skin rashes, joint pain, eye inflammation, and liver and biliary tract disease.

Another complication of colitis is the development of strictures, which are narrow areas in the colon that can obstruct the passage of stool. This can cause constipation, abdominal pain, and bloating. In some cases, surgery may be necessary to remove the strictures.

In addition to the physical complications, colitis can also have a significant impact on a person's emotional and mental well-being. Living with a chronic illness can be stressful and can lead to feelings of depression and anxiety. It's important to be aware of these emotional and mental health issues and to seek help if needed.

Colitis treatment typically includes medications to reduce inflammation, such as aminosalicylates, corticosteroids, and immunomodulators. Biologics and other newer medications are also available for more severe cases of colitis. In some cases, surgery may be necessary to remove the colon and rectum.

It's also important to maintain a healthy diet and lifestyle to manage colitis. This may include avoiding foods that can worsen symptoms, eating a diet high in fiber and nutrients, and getting regular exercise.

Living with colitis can be challenging, but with the right treatment, lifestyle changes, and support, people with colitis can lead full, active lives. It's important to work with your doctor to develop a treatment plan that's right for you and to be aware of the potential risks and complications associated with colitis.

In conclusion, Colitis is a chronic condition that causes inflammation in the lining of the colon and rectum, and it has several risks and complications associated with it. One of the most common risks associated with colitis is the development of ulcers in the colon and rectum. Another risk is the development of cancer of the colon and rectum. Colitis can also cause other complications such as malnutrition, weight loss, anemia and extra-intestinal manifestations. Strictures can also develop and surgery may be necessary to remove them.

Chapter Twenty-Four

Living with Colitis

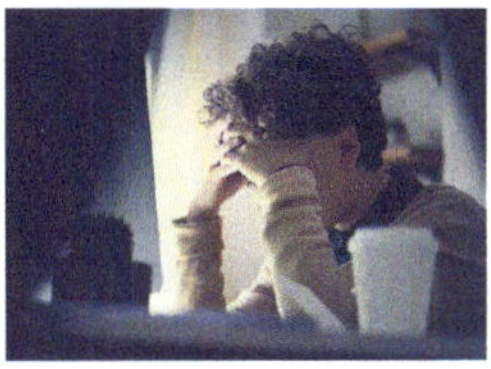

Living with colitis can be a challenging experience. Colitis is a general term used to describe inflammation of the colon, and there are several different types of colitis, each with its own set of symptoms and treatment options. Some of the most common types of colitis include ulcerative colitis, Crohn's disease, and microscopic colitis.

Ulcerative colitis is a type of inflammatory bowel disease (IBD) that causes inflammation and ulcers in the inner lining of the large intestine. Symptoms of ulcerative colitis can include abdominal pain and cramping, diarrhea, and blood in the stool.

Crohn's disease is another type of IBD that can affect any part of the digestive tract, from the mouth to the anus. Symptoms of Crohn's disease can include abdominal pain and cramping, diarrhea, weight loss, and malnutrition.

Microscopic colitis is a type of colitis that is characterized by inflammation of the colon that can only be seen under a microscope. Symptoms of microscopic colitis can include watery diarrhea, abdominal pain, and weight loss.

Living with colitis can be difficult due to the chronic nature of the condition. The symptoms can be unpredictable and can range from mild to severe. The chronic diarrhea, abdominal pain, and blood in the stool can make it difficult to maintain a normal lifestyle and can lead to feelings of isolation and depression.

Managing colitis requires a combination of medications, diet, and lifestyle changes. Medications such as aminosalicylates, corticosteroids, immunomodulators, and biologic therapies may be used to reduce inflammation and alleviate symptoms.

Dietary changes can also play a crucial role in managing colitis. It is important to eat a well-balanced diet that is high in nutrients and low in fat. Some people with colitis may need to avoid certain foods that can exacerbate their symptoms. For example, some people with ulcerative colitis may need to avoid foods high in fiber, while others may need to avoid foods high in fat.

Lifestyle changes can also help to manage the symptoms of colitis. It is important to exercise regularly and to get enough sleep. Stress can also exacerbate symptoms of colitis, so it is important to manage stress through relaxation techniques such as yoga, meditation or cognitive-behavioral therapy.

It is also important to be aware of the potential complications of colitis. Some people with colitis may be at risk for developing colon cancer. In addition, colitis can also lead to other health problems such as osteoporosis, anemia, and skin problems.

Dealing with colitis can be a daily struggle, but it is important to have a support system in place. Support groups can provide a sense of community and understanding, as well as provide a platform to share information and advice. Also, having a good relationship with your healthcare provider is important, so you can discuss your symptoms, treatment options, and any concerns you may have.

In conclusion, Living with colitis can be challenging due to the chronic nature of the condition and the unpredictability of symptoms. There are different types of colitis, each with its own set of symptoms and treatment options. Managing colitis requires a combination of medications, diet, and lifestyle changes. It's also important to be aware of the potential complications of colitis and to have a support system in place. Remember that you are not alone, and it's important to reach out for help and support when needed. With the right treatment, a healthy lifestyle, and a positive attitude, it is possible to manage colitis and live a fulfilling life.

Emma's Story

Today was a rough day with my colitis. I woke up with a stomach ache and had to rush to the bathroom with diarrhea. I felt weak and dizzy, but I had to go to work anyway. I tried to eat a light breakfast, but my stomach was too upset, so I had to skip it.

At work, I struggled to focus on my tasks as I was constantly running to the bathroom. I felt embarrassed and ashamed, as I didn't want my coworkers to know about my condition. I tried to hide my symptoms, but it was difficult as I was sweating, shaking, and feeling dehydrated.

During my lunch break, I went to the bathroom again and noticed some blood in my stool. This made me worried and anxious, as I know that bleeding can be a sign of a flare-up. I decided to call my doctor and make an appointment for the next day.

In the afternoon, I felt a bit better and managed to get some work done. However, I was still feeling weak and tired, and my stomach was making loud noises. I had to cancel my plans for the evening and go home early, as I knew that I needed rest and hydration.

Back home, I took a warm bath and tried to relax. I drank some electrolyte solution and ate some plain rice, hoping that it would help me feel better. I watched some TV and read a book, trying to distract myself from my symptoms.

Overall, it was a difficult day with my colitis. I felt frustrated and helpless, as I couldn't control my symptoms and had to cancel my plans. However, I know that I have to take care of myself and prioritize my health. Tomorrow, I'll see my doctor and hopefully get some answers and help.

Sophia

's Story

Today was a good day with my colitis. I woke up feeling well-rested and energized. I had a light breakfast of oatmeal and bananas, which didn't upset my stomach. I took my medication and supplements as usual and went to work.

At work, I was able to focus on my tasks and didn't have any urgent bathroom trips. I drank plenty of water and herbal tea throughout the day, which helped me stay hydrated and calm. I also took a short walk during my break, which helped me clear my mind and reduce stress.

During lunch, I had a salad with grilled chicken and a side of sweet potatoes. It was a balanced and nutritious meal that didn't trigger any symptoms. I also brought some snacks with me, such as almonds and apple slices, in case I got hungry later.

In the afternoon, I had a meeting with my boss and colleagues. I was able to participate actively and didn't feel self-conscious about my condition. I even shared some tips on mindfulness and stress reduction, which were well-received.

After work, I went to the gym and did some light cardio and strength training. I felt strong and capable, despite my condition. I also chatted with some fellow gym-goers, which boosted my mood and social connection.

Back home, I had a light dinner of grilled fish and steamed vegetables. I watched a movie and did some gentle yoga before bed. I felt grateful for a good day with my colitis and hopeful for more to come.

Olivia

’s Story

Today was a challenging day with my colitis. I woke up with a headache and stomach cramps, which made it difficult to get out of bed. I had some toast and tea for breakfast, but it didn't settle well.

At work, I had to run to the bathroom several times and had some urgency and diarrhea. I felt embarrassed and ashamed, as I didn't want my coworkers to hear or see me. I also had some nausea and bloating, which made it hard to focus on my tasks.

During my lunch break, I went to the nearest park and sat on a bench. I did some deep breathing and visualization exercises, trying to calm my nervous system. I also drank some ginger tea and ate a banana, hoping that it would help my digestion.

In the afternoon, I had a meeting with a client and had to postpone it due to my symptoms. I felt frustrated and disappointed, as I didn't want to let down my team or the client. I also had some joint pain and fatigue, which made me feel even more drained and achy.

After work, I went home and lay down on the couch. I watched some TV and tried to distract myself from my symptoms. I took a hot bath and used a heating pad on my lower abdomen, which provided some relief. I also drank some bone broth and ate some plain rice, hoping that it would be gentle on my gut.

Overall, it was a tough day with my colitis. I felt overwhelmed and vulnerable, as I couldn't predict or control my symptoms. However, I know that I have to be patient and kind to myself, and seek support when needed.

Mia's Story

Today, I went to the shopping mall with my friends, and it was a challenging day with my colitis. I woke up feeling okay, but I was a bit nervous about going out because I never know when my symptoms will act up. I had a light breakfast of toast and tea and took my medication as usual.

At the mall, we started shopping and browsing the stores. I was feeling okay at first, but soon after, I started feeling some cramps and urgency. I quickly excused myself and went to the bathroom. It was so uncomfortable and painful, and I couldn't stay in there for long. I came out and tried to pretend that everything was okay, but my friends could tell that I was not feeling well.

We stopped at a café for a break, and my friends ordered some food and drinks, but I couldn't eat anything because I was feeling so sick. I drank some water and tried to relax, but I was feeling anxious and embarrassed. We continued walking around the mall, but I was struggling to keep up, and I had to make several trips to the bathroom.

At one point, I had a sudden urge to go to the bathroom, and I couldn't hold it in. I was so embarrassed and ashamed, and I didn't know what to do. I quickly went to the bathroom and cleaned myself up, but I was feeling so helpless and hopeless.

I decided to go home early because I couldn't take it anymore. I said goodbye to my friends and went home. I took a warm bath and tried to relax, but I was feeling so sad and frustrated. I know that I can't control my colitis, and it's not my fault, but it's hard not to feel so helpless and ashamed.

Sophie's Story:

Today was a challenging day with my colitis. I decided to go to the shopping mall with my friends, hoping to have some fun and distraction. But it turned out to be a difficult experience.

At the mall, we started browsing the stores and trying on clothes. I was feeling okay at first, but soon after, I started feeling some cramps and urgency. I quickly excused myself and went to the bathroom. It was so uncomfortable and painful, and I couldn't stay in there for long. I came out and tried to pretend that everything was okay, but my friends could tell that I was not feeling well.

We stopped at a café for a break, and my friends ordered some food and drinks, but I couldn't eat anything because I was feeling so sick. I drank some water and tried to relax, but I was feeling anxious and embarrassed. We continued walking around the mall, but I was struggling to keep up, and I had to make several trips to the bathroom.

At one point, I had a sudden urge to go to the bathroom, and I couldn't hold it in. I was so embarrassed and ashamed, and I didn't know what to do. I quickly went to the bathroom and cleaned myself up, but I was feeling so helpless and hopeless.

I decided to go home early because I couldn't take it anymore. I said goodbye to my friends and went home. I took a warm bath and tried to relax, but I was feeling so sad and frustrated. I know that I can't control my colitis, and it's not my fault, but it's hard not to feel so helpless and ashamed.

Alex's Story:

Today was a tough day with my colitis at work. I woke up feeling okay, but as soon as I got to work, my stomach started feeling uneasy. I had some toast and tea for breakfast, but it didn't settle well.

At work, I had to run to the bathroom several times and had some urgency and diarrhea. I felt embarrassed and ashamed, as I didn't want my coworkers to hear or see me. I also had some nausea and bloating, which made it hard to focus on my tasks.

During lunch, I had a salad with grilled chicken and a side of sweet potatoes. It was a balanced and nutritious meal that didn't trigger any symptoms. I also brought some snacks with me, such as almonds and apple slices, in case I got hungry later.

In the afternoon, I had a meeting with my boss and colleagues. I was able to participate actively and didn't feel self-conscious about my condition. However, towards the end of the meeting, I had to excuse myself and go to the bathroom. I felt so embarrassed and frustrated, as I didn't want to disrupt the meeting or draw attention to myself.

After work, I went home and lay down on the couch. I watched some TV and tried to distract myself from my symptoms. I took a hot bath and used a heating pad on my lower abdomen, which provided some relief. I also drank some bone broth and ate some plain rice, hoping that it would be gentle on my gut.

Overall, it was a challenging day with my colitis at work. I felt overwhelmed and vulnerable, as I couldn't predict or control my symptoms. However, I know that I have to be patient and kind to myself, and seek support when needed.

Tom's Story:

Today was a challenging day with my colitis at the construction site. I woke up feeling okay, but as soon as I got to work, my stomach started feeling uneasy. I had some oatmeal and tea for breakfast, but it didn't settle well.

At the site, I had to run to the portable toilet several times and had some urgency and diarrhea. I felt embarrassed and ashamed, as I didn't want my coworkers to hear or see me. I also had some abdominal pain and cramps, which made it hard to focus on my tasks.

During lunch, I had a sandwich with turkey and cheese and a side of carrots. It was a balanced and nutritious meal that didn't trigger any symptoms. However, my coworkers noticed that I wasn't eating much and started making fun of me. They called me names and made jokes about my condition, which made me feel even worse.

In the afternoon, I had to work on a ladder and was feeling weak and dizzy. I had to take frequent breaks and couldn't keep up with the pace of the others. My coworkers started making fun of me again, calling me lazy and useless.

After work, I went home and lay down on the couch. I felt so sad and frustrated, as I didn't want my colitis to define me or limit me. I know that it's a chronic condition that I have to manage, but it's hard to deal with the stigma and discrimination.

I decided to talk to my supervisor and HR about my condition and the bullying I was experiencing. They were supportive and understanding, and they promised to take action against the harassers.

Overall, it was a tough day with my colitis at the construction site. I felt overwhelmed and vulnerable, as I couldn't predict or control my symptoms. However, I know that I have to be brave and stand up for myself, and seek support when needed.

Anna's

Story:

Today was a nerve-wracking day with my colitis at a job interview. I woke up feeling anxious and stressed, as I wanted to make a good impression but didn't know how my symptoms would behave. I had some toast and tea for breakfast, but it didn't settle well.

At the interview, I tried to stay calm and focused, but I was feeling some cramps and urgency. I excused myself and went to the bathroom before the interview, hoping that it would help. However, during the interview, I had to hold back my urge to go to the bathroom, which made me feel even more uncomfortable and distressed.

I tried to answer the questions as best as I could, but my mind was racing, and I couldn't concentrate. I was so worried that my condition would affect my chances of getting the job.

After the interview, I went to the bathroom again and felt some relief. I decided to take a walk in the park and do some deep breathing exercises, trying to calm my nervous system. I also drank some water and ate a banana, hoping that it would help my digestion.

Back home, I lay down on the couch and watched some TV. I felt so exhausted and drained, both physically and emotionally. I know that I have to be patient and kind to myself, and take care of my health first and foremost.

Overall, it was a challenging day with my colitis at the job interview. I felt overwhelmed and vulnerable, as I couldn't predict or control my symptoms. However, I know that I have to keep trying and believe in myself, and seek support when needed.

Jane's

Story:

Today was a great day with my colitis out with friends. I woke up feeling well-rested and energized, and I was excited to meet my friends for brunch. I had some yogurt and granola for breakfast, which didn't upset my stomach. I also took my medication and supplements as usual.

At brunch, I had a veggie omelet and a side of fruit. It was a balanced and nutritious meal that didn't trigger any symptoms. I also drank some herbal tea and chatted with my friends, feeling comfortable and relaxed.

After brunch, we went for a walk in the park and enjoyed the sunshine and fresh air. I felt so grateful for the company of my friends and the beauty of nature. We took some photos and laughed together, feeling carefree and happy.

During the walk, I had to excuse myself and go to the bathroom, but it wasn't a big deal. My friends were understanding and supportive, and they didn't make a big deal out of it. I felt so fortunate to have such kind and compassionate friends who didn't judge me for my condition.

After the walk, we went to a movie and enjoyed some popcorn and soda. I felt relaxed and comfortable, knowing that I was in good company. I also drank plenty of water and stayed hydrated, which helped my digestion and overall well-being.

Back home, I felt so proud of myself for having a great day out with friends despite my colitis. I know that it's a chronic condition that I have to manage, but it doesn't define me or limit me. I have become stronger and more resilient over time, and I know that I can overcome any challenge.

Chapter Twenty-Five

FAQ

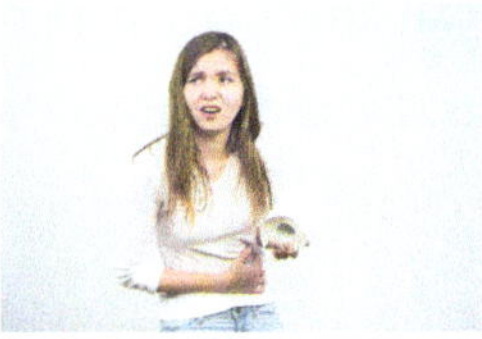

A picture containing person, standing, posing

Description automatically generated

What are the warning signs of colitis?

Most people with colitis don't experience any symptoms in the early stages of the disease. When symptoms do appear, they may come on gradually or suddenly. The most common symptom of colitis is bloody diarrhea. This can be accompanied by abdominal pain and cramping, fatigue, weight loss, and fever.

If you experience any of these symptoms, it's important to see your doctor right away so that they can diagnose and treat your condition. Left untreated, colitis can lead to serious complications, such as dehydration, malnutrition, and even death.

There are a few different types of colitis, each with its own set of symptoms. The most common types are ulcerative colitis and Crohn's disease.

Ulcerative colitis causes ulcers, or sores, to form in the lining of the rectum and colon. The ulcers may bleed and the inflammation can cause the colon to empty more frequently, resulting in diarrhea. Ulcerative colitis can also cause abdominal pain, fatigue, and weight loss.

Crohn's disease is similar to ulcerative colitis, but it can affect any part of the gastrointestinal tract from the mouth to the anus. In addition to the symptoms of ulcerative colitis, Crohn's disease can also cause mouth sores, anemia, and joint pain.

There are other, less common types of colitis that have their own sets of symptoms. These include infectious colitis, ischemic colitis, allergic colitis, and primary sclerosing cholangitis.

Infectious colitis is caused by a bacterial, viral, or parasitic infection. Symptoms include diarrhea, abdominal pain, cramping, and fever.

Ischemic colitis is caused by a lack of blood flow to the colon. Symptoms include abdominal pain, cramping, diarrhea, and Rectal bleeding.

Allergic colitis is caused by an allergic reaction to a food or medication. Symptoms include diarrhea, abdominal pain, and cramping.

Primary sclerosing cholangitis is a chronic liver disease that can cause inflammation and damage to the bile ducts. Symptoms include fatigue, itching, jaundice, and abdominal pain.

No matter what type of colitis you have, it's important to see your doctor if you experience any symptoms. Early diagnosis and treatment is essential to preventing serious complications.

Can colitis be cured?

There is no one answer to whether colitis can be cured as the condition can vary greatly from person to person. In some cases, colitis may be caused by an infection or other acute event and resolved completely with treatment. However, for others, colitis may be chronic and require long-term management.

Certain types of colitis, such as ulcerative colitis, may be treated with surgery to remove the affected portion of the colon. This can often provide symptom relief, but it is not a cure. In other cases, medication may be used to help control the inflammation associated with colitis. Some people may find that making lifestyle changes, such as avoiding trigger foods, can also help to manage their symptoms.

There is currently no cure for colitis, but treatment can often help to control the symptoms and improve quality of life. If you are living with colitis, it is important to work with your healthcare team to find the best treatment plan for you.

What are the symptoms of colitis in adults?

The symptoms of colitis differ depending on the type of colitis. However, common symptoms in adults include abdominal pain and cramping, bloating, gas, diarrhea, and weight loss. With ulcerative colitis, bleeding may also occur. The stool may be bloody or tarry.

Symptom onset may be gradual or sudden. Some people experience long periods of remission, during which they may have no symptoms. Then, symptoms may flare up for a few weeks or months, followed by another period of remission.

Different types of colitis can cause different symptoms. For example, Crohn's disease often leads to fatigue, whereas ulcerative colitis does not. Other symptoms that may occur with colitis include:

-Anemia

-Dehydration

-Fever

-Loss of appetite

-Malnutrition

-Night sweats

-Rectal bleeding

-Urinary frequency or urgency

If you experience any of these symptoms, it's important to see your doctor so they can diagnose and treat the problem. Left untreated, colitis can lead to serious complications, such as bleeding, dehydration, and malnutrition.

What Food Triggers colitis?

There is no one definitive answer to this question as everyone experiences colitis differently and what may trigger an attack for one person, may not have the same effect on another. That said, there are certain foods that are commonly known to trigger or exacerbate symptoms in those with colitis, and it is generally recommended that people with the condition avoid these trigger foods where possible.

Some of the most commonly reported trigger foods for colitis include dairy products, high fat foods, caffeine, alcohol, spicy foods, and processed foods. Many people with colitis also find that their symptoms are worse when they eat foods that are high in acidity or gluten.

Dairy products are a common trigger food for colitis as they can be difficult for the body to digest. This is because they contain a high amount of lactose, which is a sugar that is not easily broken down by the digestive system. For people with colitis, this can lead to increased bloating, gas, and abdominal pain.

High fat foods are another common trigger as they can slow down the digestive process and make it difficult for the body to absorb nutrients. This can lead to the worsening of symptoms such as diarrhea, abdominal pain, and fatigue.

Caffeine is a stimulant that can speed up the digestive process and cause diarrhea. For people with colitis, this can trigger an attack or make existing symptoms worse.

Alcohol can also irritate the digestive system and trigger symptoms such as diarrhea, abdominal pain, and nausea.

Spicy foods can cause inflammation in the digestive system and trigger symptoms such as abdominal pain, diarrhea, and vomiting.

Processed foods are often high in salt, sugar, and fat, which can all trigger symptoms in people with colitis. These foods can also be difficult to digest and may cause bloating, gas, and abdominal pain.

While there is no one definitive answer to what food triggers colitis, these are some of the most commonly reported trigger foods. It is generally recommended that people with colitis avoid these foods where possible to help manage their condition.

Is colitis very serious?

Colitis is an inflammation of the colon. It can be caused by a variety of things, including infection, poor diet, stress, and certain medications. Colitis can be a very serious condition, and it is important to see a doctor if you think you may have it.

There are a few different types of colitis, each with different symptoms and treatments. The most common type is ulcerative colitis, which usually affects the large intestine. Symptoms of ulcerative colitis can include abdominal pain, bloody diarrhea, weight loss, and fatigue. If left untreated, ulcerative colitis can lead to serious complications, such as bleeding, malnutrition, and even death.

Crohn's disease is another type of colitis that can be very serious. Crohn's disease is an inflammation of the digestive system, and it can cause a variety of symptoms, including abdominal pain, diarrhea, weight loss, and fatigue. Crohn's disease can also lead to serious complications, such as intestinal bleeding, malnutrition, and even death.

Colitis is a serious condition that should not be ignored. If you think you may have colitis, it is important to see a doctor so that you can get the proper diagnosis and treatment.

How do you make colitis go away?

There's no surefire way to make colitis go away, but there are treatments that can help lessen your symptoms and get the condition under control. The first step is to see a doctor or gastroenterologist to get a proper diagnosis. From there, they can work with you to develop a treatment plan that may include medication, diet changes, and stress-relief techniques.

Medications are the most common form of treatment for colitis. The type of medication will depend on the severity of your condition. For milder cases, over-the-counter anti-inflammatory drugs like ibuprofen may be enough to help with symptoms. For more severe cases, your doctor may prescribe stronger anti-inflammatory drugs, immune-suppressants, or antibiotics.

Diet changes can also be helpful in managing colitis. Eating smaller, more frequent meals instead of large ones can help ease gastrointestinal discomfort. You may also want to avoid problem foods that seem to trigger your symptoms. Common triggers include caffeine, alcohol, spicy foods, and dairy. Keeping a food diary can help you pinpoint which foods are problematic for you.

Finally, stress-relief techniques can be helpful in managing colitis. Stress can worsen symptoms, so finding ways to reduce stress in your life can help you feel better. relaxation techniques like meditation, yoga, and deep breathing exercises can all help to reduce stress. Some people find that regular exercise is also helpful in managing stress and colitis symptoms.

While there is no cure for colitis, there are treatments that can help manage the symptoms and provide some relief. Some people with colitis may only need occasional medical attention, while others may need to be hospitalized. With proper treatment and care, many people with colitis can lead normal, productive lives.

What is the best treatment for colitis?

The best treatment for colitis is not entirely clear, as the condition can vary greatly from person to person. However, there are a few options that seem to be effective for many people.

One option is medication. There are a number of different drugs that can be used to treat colitis, and the best one for a particular person will depend on the severity of their condition and any other health issues they may have. Some common medications used to treat colitis include corticosteroids, immune suppressants, and antibiotics.

Another option is surgery. This is usually only recommended for people with severe colitis that has not responded to other treatments. Surgery can involve removing part of the colon, or the entire colon. It can also involve other procedures, such as widening the opening of the colon, to make it easier for waste to pass through.

For many people, a combination of different treatments is the best approach. This might include medication, surgery, and lifestyle changes. Lifestyle changes that can help manage colitis include stress reduction, quitting smoking, and following a healthy diet.

Whatever treatment approach is used, it is important to work with a doctor to create a plan that is right for the individual.

What happens if you ignore colitis?

If you have colitis and do not seek treatment, the symptoms will persist and may even worsen over time. The inflammation will damage the lining of the intestines, causing bleeding and pain. In severe cases, the inflammation can lead to ulcers and perforations in the intestine. If untreated, colitis can be fatal.

What should I avoid eating with colitis?

There is no one-size-fits-all answer to this question, as everyone's experience with colitis is different. However, there are some general guidelines that can help you figure out what to avoid eating with colitis.

First, it's important to avoid any foods that trigger your colitis symptoms. Everyone's triggers are different, but common triggers include spicy food, caffeine, alcohol, and anything that is high in fat or fibre. If you're not sure what your triggers are, it can be helpful to keep a food diary to help you identify them.

Second, it's important to eat a healthy and balanced diet. This means eating plenty of fruits, vegetables, and whole grains, and limiting processed and sugary foods. Eating a healthy diet will help to reduce inflammation throughout your body, which can help to ease your colitis symptoms.

Finally, it's important to stay hydrated by drinking plenty of water. This will help to keep your digestive system working properly and can also help to reduce inflammation.

If you're unsure about what to eat with colitis, it's always best to speak to your doctor or a Registered Dietitian. They can help you create a customized plan that fits your needs and your lifestyle.

What foods help heal colitis?

There is no one-size-fits-all answer to the question of which foods help heal colitis, as the condition can vary significantly from person to person. However, there are some general tips that may be helpful for people with the condition.

Firstly, it is important to eat a healthy and balanced diet. This means eating plenty of fruits, vegetables, and whole grains, and avoiding processed foods, sugary snacks, and excessive amounts of saturated and unhealthy fats.

People with colitis may also find it helpful to eat smaller, more frequent meals rather than three large meals each day. This can help to reduce the amount of strain on the digestive system.

There are also a number of specific foods that may help to ease the symptoms of colitis. These include probiotic-rich foods such as yogurt and sauerkraut, as well as anti-inflammatory foods such as omega-3 fatty acids, turmeric, and ginger.

Of course, it is important to speak to a doctor or qualified healthcare professional before making any major changes to diet or lifestyle. They will be able to offer tailored advice based on the individual's specific situation.

How long does colitis usually last?

Colitis refers to a chronic inflammation of the large intestine, specifically the colon. The inflammation is characterized by ulcers in the inner lining of the colon, which can lead to a range of symptoms, including abdominal pain, bloody stool, and weight loss. The exact cause of colitis is unknown, but it is believed to be the result of a combination of genetic and environmental factors.

Colitis is a chronic condition, which means that it can last for months or even years. The length of time that a person experiences colitis will vary depending on the severity of their condition. For some people, colitis may only last for a few weeks or months, while for others it may be a lifelong condition. There is no cure for colitis, but there are treatments available that can help to manage the symptoms and improve the quality of life for those affected by the condition.

How is colitis diagnosed?

Your doctor will ask you about your symptoms and medical history. They will also give you a physical exam. Tests that may be done include:

-a stool sample to look for blood or parasites

-a colonoscopy or sigmoidoscopy to check for inflammation and ulcers in the large intestine

-a barium enema to check for blockages or problems with the shape of the large intestine

-a CT scan or MRI to check for abscesses, fistulas, or other problems

Your doctor may also do tests to rule out other conditions, such as irritable bowel syndrome or Crohn's disease.

Is yogurt good for colitis?

There is some evidence that consuming yogurt may help to ease the symptoms of colitis. Colitis is a condition that causes inflammation of the colon and can lead to a number of uncomfortable symptoms, including abdominal pain and cramping, diarrhea, and bloating. Some research suggests that the beneficial bacteria found in yogurt may help to reduce inflammation in the gut and improve gut health, which may in turn help to ease the symptoms of colitis.

That said, it is important to remember that yogurt is not a cure for colitis and more research is needed to confirm its effectiveness. Additionally, yogurt may not be suitable for everyone with colitis - for example, those who are lactose intolerant may find that yogurt worsens their symptoms. If you are considering trying yogurt as a way to ease your colitis symptoms, it is important to speak to your doctor first to ensure that it is the right option for you.

While there is no cure for colitis, many treatments are available to help manage the condition. With proper medical care and treatment, most people with colitis can lead normal, active lives.

Is colitis worse than Crohn's?

There are two main types of inflammatory bowel disease (IBD): Crohn's disease and ulcerative colitis. Both of these conditions can be painful and debilitating, but patients often debate which one is worse. In reality, there is no clear answer because each person experiences IBD differently. Some people may find that ulcerative colitis is more disruptive to their life while others may feel that Crohn's disease is more severe.

Both Crohn's disease and ulcerative colitis are chronic conditions that cause inflammation in the gastrointestinal tract. The inflammation can lead to a number of symptoms including abdominal pain, diarrhea, weight loss, and fatigue. The severity of these symptoms can vary from person to person. Some people may only experience occasional mild flare-ups while others may have constant, debilitating symptoms.

There is no cure for either Crohn's disease or ulcerative colitis, but there are treatments available that can help to manage the symptoms. Some people with IBD may only require occasional medication or lifestyle changes to keep their symptoms under control. Others may need more aggressive treatment, such as surgery, to control their disease.

Some people may find that Crohn's disease is more difficult to manage because it can affect any part of the gastrointestinal tract. This can make it more difficult to find treatments that are effective. Ulcerative colitis, on the other hand, only affects the large intestine. This means that there are usually more treatment options available.

Ultimately, there is no clear answer to whether Crohn's disease or ulcerative colitis is worse. Each person experiences IBD differently and what may be a minor annoyance for one person could be a major issue for another. If you are living with IBD, it is important to work with your doctor to find a treatment plan that works for you.

Can stress cause colitis?

Stress is a common trigger for acute episodes of ulcerative colitis (UC), and may also play a role in disease flares and remission. While the exact mechanism is unknown, stress may alter the gut microbiota, increase inflammation, or affect the gut-brain axis. Although stress does not cause UC, managing stress may help to prevent flares and improve quality of life.

There are many different ways to manage stress, and what works for one person may not work for another. Some helpful stress-management techniques include exercise, relaxation techniques such as deep breathing or meditation, journaling, and spending time in nature. In addition, talking to a therapist or counselor can provide support and skills to help manage stress.

Will colitis go away on its own?

There is no one answer to this question as it varies from person to person. For some, colitis may go away on its own, while for others it may be a chronic condition that requires lifelong management. The general consensus is that colitis is a serious condition that should not be ignored, and that seeking professional medical help is the best course of action.

left unchecked, colitis can lead to serious complications such as dehydration, malnutrition, and even life-threatening conditions such as sepsis. In some cases, surgery may be required to remove part of the colon that is affected by colitis. Seeking early medical treatment is crucial in managing colitis and preventing these complications.

If you are experiencing any symptoms of colitis, it is important to see a doctor as soon as possible. They will be able to diagnose your condition and develop a treatment plan that is right for you.

How many times a day do you poop with colitis?

For people with colitis, 'normal' bowel movements can range anywhere from a couple of times a day to a couple of times a week. The key is listening to your body and knowing what's 'normal' for you.

There's no magic number of times you should be pooping each day, but most people with colitis generally fall somewhere in the range of 3 to 5 times a day. This means that, on average, you're pooping about once every 3 to 4 hours.

Of course, this is just a general guideline. Some people with colitis may poop more or less often than this. And it's not unusual for your 'normal' to change over time. For example, you may find that your bowel movements are more frequent during a flare-up, and then return to normal (or close to normal) during periods of remission.

If you're concerned about how often you're pooping, or if you're experiencing any other symptoms like pain, bleeding, or diarrhea, it's always best to check in with your doctor. They can help figure out what's going on and offer treatments to get your bowel movements back on track.

How often do you poop with colitis?

There's no one answer to this question since everyone experiences colitis differently. However, it's generally accepted that people with colitis may have more frequent bowel movements than people without the condition. This is because the inflammation in the colon can cause diarrhea.

How often you poop with colitis really depends on the severity of your symptoms. Some people may go to the bathroom several times a day while others may only go a few times a week. There may be days when you have several bowel movements in quick succession, followed by days with no bowel movements at all.

The severity of your symptoms may also fluctuate. For example, you may find that your symptoms are worse after eating certain foods or during times of stress. You may have periods of remission where your symptoms seem to disappear altogether, only to have them flare up again at a later date.

If you're concerned about how often you're pooping, or if you're experiencing other symptoms like abdominal pain, blood in your stool, or weight loss, it's important to see a doctor. They can assess your individual situation and offer treatment to help control your symptoms.

Where is colitis pain felt?

Pain from colitis is felt in the lower left side of the abdomen, where the colon is located. The pain may be crampy and come and go, or it may be constant. Some people also have rectal pain and bleeding. The pain may get worse after eating, during a bowel movement, or when you lie down.

What drinks to avoid with colitis?

If you're living with colitis, it's important to be aware of the types of drinks that can trigger flares or make your symptoms worse. Some of the worst offenders include alcoholic beverages, caffeinated drinks, and sugary beverages.

Alcoholic drinks can irritate the lining of your digestive tract, making symptoms like stomach pain, diarrhea, and rectal bleeding worse. If you're struggling with colitis, it's best to avoid alcohol altogether.

Caffeinated drinks like coffee, tea, and soda can also aggravate colitis symptoms. They can stimulate your intestine and make diarrhea worse. Caffeinated beverages can also dehydrate you, which can make other colitis symptoms, like fatigue, worse.

Sugary drinks are thought to contribute to colitis flares by feeding the bad bacteria in your gut. If you have colitis, it's best to avoid sugary sodas, sports drinks, and fruit juices.

While there are some drinks that you should avoid if you have colitis, there are also some that can help ease your symptoms. water is always a good choice, as it will help keep you hydrated. Herbal tea can also be soothing, and some people find that probiotic drinks help alleviate colitis symptoms.

Colitis is a serious condition that can lead to long-term health problems. If you think you may have colitis, it is important to see a doctor right away.

How do I know if I have IBS or ulcerative colitis?

If you have any symptoms of IBS or ulcerative colitis, it is important to see a doctor to get a diagnosis. There are some key differences between the two conditions that can help your doctor make a diagnosis.

IBS is a disorder of the gastrointestinal tract that can cause a range of symptoms including abdominal pain, bloating, diarrhea, and constipation. IBS is a chronic condition that can last for months or years. There is no known cure for IBS, but there are treatments that can help relieve symptoms.

Ulcerative colitis is a chronic inflammatory bowel disease that affects the colon and rectum. Ulcerative colitis can cause a range of symptoms including abdominal pain, diarrhea, fatigue, and weight loss. Ulcerative colitis is a serious condition that can lead to life-threatening complications. There is no known cure for ulcerative colitis, but there are treatments that can help manage the symptoms.

There are some key differences between IBS and ulcerative colitis that can help your doctor make a diagnosis. IBS is a chronic condition that can last for months or years, while ulcerative colitis is a serious condition that can lead to life-threatening complications. IBS can cause a range of symptoms including abdominal pain, bloating, diarrhea, and constipation, while ulcerative colitis can cause a range of symptoms including abdominal pain, diarrhea, fatigue, and weight loss. There is no known cure for either condition, but there are treatments that can help manage symptoms.

Does colitis always show up on colonoscopy?

No, colitis does not always show up on colonoscopy. Many people with colitis do not have any symptoms and are unaware that they have the condition. When symptoms do present, they can vary greatly from person to person, making it difficult to diagnose. Colonoscopy is often used as a diagnostic tool for colitis, but it is not always conclusive. In some cases, other tests, such as biopsies, may be necessary to confirm a diagnosis.

How do you test for ulcerative colitis?

There are a few different ways that doctors can test for ulcerative colitis. One way is through a colonoscopy. This is where a doctor inserts a long, thin tube with a camera on the end into the patient's rectum and then up into their colon. This allows the doctor to see the inside of the colon and look for any ulcers or swelling.

Another way to test for ulcerative colitis is through a sigmoidoscopy. This is similar to a colonoscopy, but the tube only goes into the patient's rectum and lower part of their colon.

Blood tests can also be used to help diagnose ulcerative colitis. These tests can look for things like anemia, which can be caused by bleeding from the ulcers in the colon. They can also look for inflammation markers in the blood, which can be a sign of inflammation in the colon.

A biopsy is another way to test for ulcerative colitis. This is where a small sample of tissue is taken from the colon and looked at under a microscope. This can help to confirm the diagnosis of ulcerative colitis and rule out other potential causes of the symptoms.

What are 3 common complications of someone with ulcerative colitis?

If you have ulcerative colitis (UC), you're likely always on the lookout for potential complications. While UC can be a lifelong disease with no cure, most people who have it are able to manage their symptoms and live relatively normal lives. Still, UC can lead to some serious complications, some of which can be life-threatening.

Bloody diarrhea is one of the most common and most serious complications of UC. The inflammation in your colon can cause your colon to bleed, and this can lead to anemia.

Another common complication of UC is malnutrition. This can happen because the inflammation in your colon can make it difficult for your body to absorb nutrients from food. Additionally, chronic diarrhea can lead to dehydration, which can also cause malnutrition.

UC can also lead to an increased risk of colon cancer. This is because the inflammation in your colon can cause changes in the cells that line your colon, which can lead to cancer. People with UC are typically screened for colon cancer more frequently than people without UC.

While these are some of the most common complications of UC, they are by no means the only ones. Other potential complications include osteoporosis, kidney stones, gallstones, and liver disease. It's important to work with your doctor to manage your UC and to monitor for any potential complications.

What drinks soothe colitis?

There are many different drinks that can help soothe colitis. Some people find that chamomile tea or green tea can be helpful in soothing their symptoms. You can also try adding some ginger to your diet, either in tea or in food. Some people find that probiotics can also help, so you might want to try yogurt or kombucha. There are many different options to explore, so talk to your doctor or dietitian to see what might work best for you.

What foods worsen ulcerative colitis?

If you have ulcerative colitis, you may have to pay attention to the foods you eat. Some foods can make your symptoms worse.

When you have ulcerative colitis, the lining of your colon becomes inflamed. This can cause abdominal pain and cramping, diarrhea, and bleeding. Eating certain foods can make these symptoms worse.

spicy foods

high-fat foods

processed foods

caffeine

alcohol

Spicy foods can cause abdominal pain and diarrhea. Fatty foods can make diarrhea worse. Processed foods can contain chemicals that can irritate your colon. Caffeine and alcohol can also make symptoms worse.

If you have ulcerative colitis, you may need to avoid these foods or eat them in moderation. You should talk to your doctor about what type of diet is best for you.

Is colitis worse than IBS?

This is a difficult question to answer, as it depends on the individual. Some people may find that colitis is a more debilitating and severe condition than IBS, while others may find that IBS is more disruptive to their everyday life. Ultimately, it is up to the individual to decide which condition is more bothersome or severe.

Both colitis and IBS are chronic gastrointestinal disorders that can cause a great deal of discomfort and disruption to one's life. Colitis is characterized by inflammation of the colon, which can lead to cramping, diarrhea, and bloody stools. IBS, on the other hand, is a disorder that affects the way the digestive system works, and can cause bloating, constipation, and abdominal pain.

While both conditions can be very troublesome, there are some key differences between them. Colitis is often more severe, as it can lead to life-threatening complications such as bleeding and dehydration. In addition, colitis tends to be more chronic, meaning that it can last for months or even years, while IBS may come and go over time.

So, is colitis worse than IBS? It really depends on the individual. Some people may find that colitis is more debilitating, while others may find that IBS is more disruptive. Ultimately, it is up to the individual to decide which condition is more bothersome or severe.

There is no one-size-fits-all answer to the question of how to treat colitis, as the condition can vary greatly from person to person. However, some general tips on how to manage the condition include eating a healthy diet, avoiding triggers, and keeping a regular bathroom schedule. Medications can also be used to help control inflammation and pain. Ultimately, working with a healthcare team to develop a personalized treatment plan is the best way to manage colitis.

How often do you need a colonoscopy if you have ulcerative colitis?

If you have ulcerative colitis, you'll need to have a colonoscopy every one to two years. This will help your doctor check for any changes in your colon and to rule out cancer.

What is the peak age for ulcerative colitis?

Most people with ulcerative colitis are diagnosed between the ages of 15 and 30. However, the disease can occur at any age. Ulcerative colitis is more common in men than in women. The peak age for ulcerative colitis is 35.

Ulcerative colitis is a chronic inflammation of the large intestine, also known as the colon. The colon is the last part of the digestive tract. Ulcerative colitis usually affects the innermost lining of the colon, where ulcers form. Ulcerative colitis is different from Crohn's disease, another type of inflammatory bowel disease, because it only affects the large intestine. Ulcerative colitis can also affect the rectum.

Ulcerative colitis is a serious condition that can be debilitating and even life-threatening. The symptoms of ulcerative colitis can vary, depending on the severity of the inflammation. Some people with ulcerative colitis have mild symptoms, while others may have more severe symptoms.

The most common symptom of ulcerative colitis is abdominal pain. Other common symptoms include diarrhea, bloody stools, weight loss, and fatigue. Some people with ulcerative colitis also experience joint pain, eye problems, and liver disease.

Ulcerative colitis is a chronic condition, which means it can last for months or years. The inflammation can come and go. When the inflammation is active, it is called a flare-up. Flare-ups can be mild, moderate, or severe. During a flare-up, symptoms may get worse. Between flare-ups, symptoms may go away completely.

Can I live a normal life with ulcerative colitis?

Ulcerative colitis (UC) is a chronic, remitting-relapsing, inflammatory bowel disease (IBD) that is characterized by mucosal ulceration in the colon and rectum. The course of the disease is variable, and patients may have symptom-free periods interspersed with flares of disease activity. The goals of medical therapy are to induce and maintain remission, prevent relapses, and improve the quality of life.

Most patients with UC can achieve disease control with medical therapy and can expect to have a normal life span. However, UC is a chronic disease that requires lifelong treatment. The disease can be associated with significant morbidity, and patients may experience episodes of flares or remission.

The cornerstone of medical therapy for UC is corticosteroids. These agents are effective in inducing remission, but they are associated with significant side effects. Furthermore, they are not effective in maintaining remission. Other medical therapies that have been shown to be effective in UC include 5-aminosalicylates, immunomodulators, and biologic agents.

The decision to initiate medical therapy for UC should be individualized based on the severity of the disease, the patient's symptoms, and the patient's preferences. Medical therapy should be initiated promptly in patients with active disease to prevent further tissue damage. In patients with mild disease, a "wait and see" approach may be taken. In general, most patients will require lifelong medical therapy to maintain disease control.

patients with UC can expect to have a normal life span. With the right medical therapy, most patients can achieve disease control and live a normal life.

What are 5 symptoms of Crohn's disease?

Crohn's disease is a chronic inflammatory disorder of the gastrointestinal tract. The most common symptoms of Crohn's disease are abdominal pain and cramping, diarrhea, weight loss, and fatigue. Other symptoms may include rectal bleeding, fevers, mouth ulcers, and skin rashes.

Crohn's disease often leads to inflammation of the intestines, which can cause a variety of symptoms. The main symptom of Crohn's disease is abdominal pain and cramping, which is usually worse after eating. This can lead to diarrhea, as well as weight loss and fatigue. Other symptoms may include rectal bleeding, fevers, mouth ulcers, and skin rashes.

Crohn's disease can be a difficult condition to manage, but there are treatments available that can help control the symptoms. If you are experiencing any of the above symptoms, please see your doctor for a diagnosis.

What are the early warning signs of Crohn's disease?

The early warning signs of Crohn's disease can be difficult to identify because they may be similar to other gastrointestinal disorders. However, there are some key symptoms that may point to Crohn's disease.

abdominal pain, cramping, and bloating

diarrhea

weight loss

fatigue

loss of appetite

anemia

blood in the stool

mouth sores

skin rash or lesions

joint pain

eye inflammation

If you experience any of these symptoms, it is important to see a doctor to get a proper diagnosis. Crohn's disease is a serious condition that can lead to debilitating consequences if not treated properly.

How serious is Crohn's disease?

Crohn's disease is an inflammatory bowel disease (IBD) that can cause severe symptoms and complications. While there is no cure for Crohn's disease, it is possible to manage the symptoms and keep the disease under control.

Crohn's disease is a chronic condition, which means it can last for months or years. The symptoms of Crohn's disease can vary, and may come and go. Some people with Crohn's disease have long periods of remission, where they have few or no symptoms. Other people may have frequent flares, where their symptoms are severe and come on suddenly.

Crohn's disease can be serious and even life-threatening. Complications of Crohn's disease include:

* Infections: Crohn's disease can cause infections in the digestive tract. These infections can be serious, and may even require hospitalization.

* Malnutrition: Crohn's disease can make it difficult to absorb nutrients from food. This can lead to malnutrition, which can be serious, and even life-threatening.

* Inflammation: Crohn's disease can cause inflammation throughout the body. This can lead to a number of serious complications, including joint pain, skin rashes, and eye problems.

* Cancer: Crohn's disease can slightly increase your risk of developing colon cancer.

While there is no cure for Crohn's disease, it is possible to manage the symptoms and keep the disease under control. Treatment for Crohn's disease can include medication, surgery, and lifestyle changes.

How do people cope with Crohn's disease?

People with Crohn's disease often have to deal with a lot of pain and other symptoms that can make everyday activities difficult. There are a number of ways that people can cope with the disease and manage their symptoms.

There are a number of medications that can help to manage the symptoms of Crohn's disease. These can include anti-inflammatory drugs, immunosuppressants, and antibiotics. People with Crohn's disease may also need to take supplements to help them absorb nutrients properly.

Surgery is sometimes necessary to treat Crohn's disease. This can involve removing part of the intestine, or other procedures.

Diet is also important for people with Crohn's disease. There are a number of foods that can trigger symptoms, so it is important to avoid these. People with Crohn's disease may also need to take special enzymes to help them digest food properly.

Exercise can also help people with Crohn's disease to manage their symptoms. Exercise can help to reduce inflammation and help the body to better cope with stress.

Psychological support can also be important for people with Crohn's disease. This can help people to deal with the stress and anxiety that can come with the disease.

In conclusion, colitis is a serious condition that can have a major impact on a person's life. While there is no cure, there are treatments available that can help control the symptoms and improve the quality of life for those affected by the condition. With proper medical care and support, people with colitis can lead happy and healthy lives.

Can I drink alcohol with colitis?

People with colitis may wonder if they can drink alcohol. There is no simple answer to this question. Some people with colitis can drink alcohol without any problems. For others, alcohol can make their symptoms worse.

If you have colitis, you should talk to your doctor about whether it is safe for you to drink alcohol. Some people with mild colitis may be able to drink alcohol in moderation. However, people with more severe colitis may need to avoid alcohol altogether.

There is some evidence that drinking alcohol can make colitis worse. Alcohol can irritate the digestive system and make inflammation worse. Drinking too much alcohol can also lead to dehydration, which can make colitis symptoms worse.

If you do decide to drink alcohol, it is important to be aware of the signs that your colitis is getting worse. If you experience more frequent or severe bouts of diarrhea, abdominal pain, or fatigue, you should stop drinking and see your doctor.

It is also important to be aware that some medications used to treat colitis can interact with alcohol. If you are taking medications for your colitis, you should talk to your doctor about whether it is safe for you to drink alcohol.

In general, it is best to limit or avoid alcohol if you have colitis. If you do drink, it is important to be aware of how your body reacts and to know the signs that your colitis is getting worse.

Do you poop a lot with colitis?

Yes, you may poop a lot with colitis. In fact, diarrhea is a common symptom of colitis. Diarrhea is defined as having three or more loose or watery stools per day. This can obviously be quite disruptive to your life. Some people with colitis may have stool that is bloody. This can be a sign that the colitis is active and you should see your doctor.

People with colitis may also experience other symptoms like abdominal pain and cramping, fatigue, weight loss, and fever. The severity of these symptoms can vary from person to person. Some people may only have mild symptoms while others may have severe symptoms that require hospitalization.

If you have colitis, it is important to see your doctor so they can make sure you are receiving the proper treatment. There are many different treatments available that can help to lessen your symptoms and even put your colitis into remission.

Will a blood test show colitis?

A blood test can show if you have colitis, but it can't diagnose the type of colitis you have. The test can also show if you have inflammation in your blood vessels.

Blood tests can show if you have a high white blood cell count, which can indicate inflammation. A high red blood cell count may indicate bleeding in the intestine. And a high platelet count may indicate that the inflammation is severe.

If you have colitis, your doctor may also order a stool sample test to look for blood in your stool.

Does colitis start suddenly?

Colitis is an inflammation of the lining of the colon. It can be acute, meaning it starts suddenly and lasts for a short time, or chronic, meaning it lasts for a long time. Acute colitis usually starts with cramps, abdominal pain, bloating, gas, and diarrhea. These symptoms may last for a few days to a week. If you have chronic colitis, you may have these symptoms for weeks or months at a time, with periods of remission in between.

There is no one cause of colitis. It can be caused by an infection, a reaction to medication, or an underlying autoimmune or inflammatory condition. Infections that can cause colitis include viruses, bacteria, and parasites. Medications that can cause colitis include nonsteroidal anti-inflammatory drugs (NSAIDs), antibiotics, and bisphosphonates. Autoimmune and inflammatory conditions that can cause colitis include Crohn's disease, ulcerative colitis, and irritable bowel syndrome (IBS).

If you have acute colitis, you will likely be treated with a course of antibiotics if an infection is the cause. If an infection is not the cause, you may be treated with NSAIDs or steroids. If you have chronic colitis, you will likely be treated with long-term NSAIDs or steroids. If you have Crohn's disease or ulcerative colitis, you may be treated with immunosuppressants. If you have IBS, you may be treated with dietary changes, medication, or both.

What is the best breakfast for colitis?

There is no one definitive answer to the question of what the best breakfast is for colitis. However, there are some things that people with colitis should keep in mind when choosing a breakfast.

Colitis is a condition that affects the large intestine and can cause symptoms like abdominal pain, diarrhea, and blood in the stool. Some people with colitis also experience fatigue, weight loss, and malnutrition. Because of this, it is important for people with colitis to make sure that their breakfast is nutritious and will give them the energy they need to get through the day.

Some people with colitis find that a high-fiber breakfast is helpful in managing their symptoms. Foods that are high in fiber include fruits, vegetables, whole grains, and beans. These foods can help to regulate the bowels and prevent diarrhea.

Fatty foods can be hard to digest for people with colitis, and may make symptoms worse. For this reason, it is often recommended that people with colitis avoid fatty foods, or at least limit their intake.

Dairy products can also be difficult to digest for people with colitis. Some people find that they can tolerate yogurt or cheese, but milk and ice cream are often more difficult to digest.

There are many different breakfast foods that can be helpful for people with colitis. Some people find that oatmeal, eggs, or toast are easy to digest and provide the nutrients they need. Others find that fruit, vegetables, or protein shakes are helpful. The important thing is to experiment to find what works best for you.

Is milk OK for colitis?

Most people with colitis can drink milk without any problems. Milk is actually a good source of calcium, which is important for people with colitis because they may be at risk for osteoporosis.

Some people with colitis may have trouble digesting lactose, the sugar found in milk. This is because they may have less lactase, the enzyme that helps digest lactose. If you have trouble digesting lactose, you can try drinking lactose-free milk or taking lactase pills before you drink milk. You can also try other calcium-rich foods, such as yogurt or cheese.

If you have severe colitis, you may need to avoid milk and other dairy products. This is because dairy products can contain high levels of fat, which can make your colitis worse.

Is colitis cancerous?

When someone is diagnosed with colitis, one of the first questions they often have is whether or not the condition is cancerous. The good news is that, in most cases, colitis is not cancerous.

There are two main types of colitis: ulcerative colitis and Crohn's disease. Both ulcerative colitis and Crohn's disease are chronic, lifelong conditions that can greatly impact a person's quality of life. Ulcerative colitis affects the large intestine (colon) and Crohn's disease can affect any part of the gastrointestinal tract, from the mouth to the anus.

While ulcerative colitis and Crohn's disease share many similarities, there are some important differences. Crohn's disease is more likely to be associated with complications such as fistulas (abnormal openings between different organs or body cavities) and abscesses (collections of pus). Crohn's disease is also more likely to lead to intestinal blockages.

Ulcerative colitis, on the other hand, is more likely to be associated with bleeding from the rectum and changes in bathroom habits. Ulcerative colitis is also the type of colitis that may be linked to an increased risk of colon cancer.

While the vast majority of people with colitis will not go on to develop colon cancer, it is important to be aware of the potential link. People with ulcerative colitis have a slightly higher risk of developing colon cancer than the general population. The risk of developing colon cancer increases with the severity of the colitis and the length of time a person has had the condition.

The good news is that, even though there is a small increased risk of developing colon cancer, the vast majority of people with colitis will never develop the disease. In fact, with early detection and treatment, the survival rate for colon cancer is quite high.

If you have been diagnosed with colitis, it is important to talk to your doctor about the best way to manage your condition. There are many effective treatments available, and the earlier the condition is detected and treated, the better the outcome is likely to be.

There is no one-size-fits-all answer to the question of how to treat colitis, as the condition can vary greatly from person to person. However, some commonly recommended treatments include dietary changes, probiotics, and medications. In some cases, surgery may also be necessary. Ultimately, the best course of action for each individual will depend on the severity of their symptoms and the underlying cause of their colitis.

How serious is infectious colitis?

Infectious colitis is a serious inflammation of the inner lining of the colon. It is usually caused by bacteria, but can also be caused by viruses, fungi, and parasites. Infectious colitis can be life-threatening if not treated promptly and properly.

The most common symptom of infectious colitis is watery diarrhea. Other symptoms may include abdominal pain, cramping, bloody stools, fever, and weight loss. If you experience any of these symptoms, it is important to see a doctor immediately.

Infectious colitis is usually treated with antibiotics. However, in some cases, hospitalization may be necessary. If the infection is severe, you may need to be given fluids and nutrition through an IV. In rare cases, surgery may be necessary to remove the infected portion of the colon.

Most people who are treated for infectious colitis make a full recovery. However, some people may experience long-term complications, such as chronic diarrhea, abdominal pain, and weight loss. If you have infectious colitis, it is important to follow your doctor's instructions and to make sure that you finish all of your antibiotics.

Can infective colitis be cured?

There are a number of different types of colitis, each with their own unique set of symptoms and causes. Infective colitis is one type of colitis, and it is caused by an infection in the colon. The most common cause of infective colitis is the bacterium Clostridium difficile, which is found in the gut. Infective colitis can also be caused by other bacteria, viruses, or parasites.

Infective colitis is usually treated with antibiotics, and most people will make a full recovery. However, some people may experience recurrent bouts of infective colitis, and a small number of people will develop a chronic form of the condition. There is no cure for chronic infective colitis, but treatments are available to help manage the symptoms.

How long does it take to get over infectious colitis?

The length of time it takes to recover from infectious colitis varies depending on the severity of the infection and the overall health of the individual. Mild cases of infectious colitis may clear up within a week, while more severe cases may take several weeks or even longer to resolve.

Infectious colitis is a type of inflammation of the colon, or large intestine, that is caused by a bacterial, viral, or parasitic infection. The most common symptom of infectious colitis is watery, bloody diarrhea. Other symptoms may include abdominal pain, cramping, nausea, vomiting, and fever.

Most cases of infectious colitis are treated with antibiotics, which are typically effective in clearing up the infection. In more severe cases, hospitalization may be necessary to treat dehydration and other complications.

Individuals with infectious colitis should drink plenty of fluids to stay hydrated and help flush the infection from their system. They should also avoid foods that may aggravate the symptoms, such as spicy or high-fat foods. Those who have severe diarrhea or vomiting may need to be hospitalized so that they can be monitored and receive intravenous fluids.

Most people recover from infectious colitis without any lasting effects. However, some individuals may experience recurrent episodes or develop a chronic form of the condition.

What are the symptoms of infectious colitis?

Infectious colitis refers to an inflammation of the large intestine (colon) that is caused by an infection. The most common cause of infectious colitis is a bacterial infection, but it can also be caused by a virus, parasite, or yeast. Infectious colitis can be mild, moderate, or severe, and can sometimes lead to life-threatening complications.

The most common symptom of infectious colitis is watery diarrhea. Diarrhea is defined as three or more loose or watery stools per day. Other symptoms of infectious colitis may include abdominal cramping, bloating, gas, nausea, vomiting, fever, and blood in the stool. Infectious colitis typically lasts for several days, and most people recover without any lasting effects. However, some people may experience severe complications, such as dehydration, sepsis, and blood poisoning.

Infectious colitis is usually diagnosed based on symptoms and a physical examination. Your doctor may also order a stool culture to test for the presence of bacteria, viruses, or parasites. Treatment for infectious colitis typically involves antibiotics to clear the infection. You may also need to take medication to relieve symptoms, such as diarrhea. In severe cases, you may need to be hospitalized for supportive care.

How is infectious colitis diagnosed?

Infectious colitis is diagnosed by testing a sample of stool for the presence of bacteria or other infectious agents. Your doctor may also order blood tests and imaging tests to rule out other causes of your symptoms.

If you have bloody diarrhea, your doctor will likely test your stool for the presence of white blood cells. White blood cells are a sign of infection. Imaging tests, such as an abdominal CT scan or an abdominal x-ray, may also be ordered to look for evidence of inflammation in your digestive tract.

Your doctor may also recommend a colonoscopy to evaluate the health of your large intestine. During a colonoscopy, a long, flexible tube is inserted into your rectum and passed through your large intestine. This allows your doctor to directly visualize the lining of your intestine and look for signs of infection or inflammation.

In some cases, a biopsy may be taken during a colonoscopy. A biopsy is a small sample of tissue that is removed from your intestine and examined under a microscope. This can provide more information about the type of infection or inflammation present in your digestive tract.

What triggers colitis?

Colitis is a chronic inflammation of the inner lining of the colon. The most common form of colitis is ulcerative colitis, which is characterized by ulcers, or sores, in the colon. Colitis can also be caused by a bacterial or viral infection, or by a reaction to a medication.

The exact cause of colitis is unknown, but it is thought to be related to an autoimmune reaction, in which the body's immune system attacks the cells of the colon. This theory is supported by the fact that colitis is more common in people with other autoimmune diseases, such as rheumatoid arthritis, celiac disease, and Crohn's disease.

genetics may also play a role in the development of colitis. Studies have shown that colitis is more common in people with certain genetic markers, such as the HLA-B27 gene.

There are also environmental factors that may contribute to the development of colitis. Stress, for example, has been shown to trigger flares in people with the condition. And, while colitis can occur at any age, it is most commonly diagnosed in people between the ages of 15 and 30.

What foods trigger colitis?

There is no one definitive answer to this question as different people can have different triggers. However, there are some common triggers that many people with colitis find helpful to avoid. These include spicy foods, caffeine, alcohol, dairy products, and processed foods. Everyone is different, so it is important to pay attention to your own body and figure out what works for you.

Spicy foods are a common trigger for colitis flares. If you find that spicy foods make your symptoms worse, it is best to avoid them. Caffeine is also a trigger for many people. Coffee, tea, and soda can all make colitis symptoms worse. Alcohol can also be a trigger. Many people with colitis find that their symptoms are worse after drinking alcohol. Dairy products can also trigger colitis flares. For some people, dairy products make their symptoms worse. Others find that they can tolerate dairy products just fine. However, it is still a good idea to avoid dairy if you can. Processed foods are also a trigger for many people. Processed foods are foods that have been chemically treated or altered in some way. They often contain a lot of sugar, salt, and fat, which can all trigger colitis flares.

If you have colitis, it is important to pay attention to your diet and figure out what works for you. Some people find that they can eat anything they want without any problems. Others find that they need to be more careful about what they eat. There is no wrong way to eat if you have colitis, as long as you are paying attention to your body and your symptoms.

As more research is conducted, the causes of colitis remain largely unknown. However, doctors have ruled out some possible causes, such as food allergies, viral infections, and parasites. The most likely cause of colitis is an overactive immune system response to a trigger, such as bacteria. Treatment for colitis generally includes medications to reduce inflammation and suppress the immune system. In severe cases, surgery may be necessary to remove part of the colon. With treatment, most people with colitis can manage their symptoms and live normal, active lives.

What foods should be avoided with colitis?

There is no one-size-fits-all answer to this question, as the best diet for someone with colitis will vary depending on the individual's specific condition. However, there are certain foods that are generally considered to be triggers for colitis flare-ups, and so it is generally advised that these be avoided.

Some common food triggers for colitis include spicy foods, high-fat foods, caffeine, alcohol, and processed foods. Foods that are high in fibre may also trigger symptoms in some people with colitis, though others find that a high-fibre diet helps to reduce symptoms.

It is important to experiment to see what works for you and to talk to a doctor or dietitian if you are unsure about what to eat.

How hard is it to live with colitis?

Colitis is an inflammation of the large intestine, specifically the colon. The colon is the final section of the digestive tract where the body stores waste until it is eliminated. When the colon becomes inflamed, it can cause a range of symptoms including abdominal pain, cramping, bloody stool, diarrhea, and weight loss. In severe cases, colitis can lead to life-threatening complications.

Living with colitis can be extremely difficult. The symptoms can be debilitating, and the constant worry about flare-ups can be exhausting. Many people with colitis are afraid to eat for fear of triggering a flare-up. This can lead to weight loss and a lack of nutrition. It can be hard to maintain a normal social life, as always having to be close to a bathroom can be embarrassing. flares can also be unpredictable, making it difficult to plan ahead.

While there is no cure for colitis, there are treatments that can help to manage the symptoms and prevent flare-ups. These include medication, dietary changes, and stress reduction. Some people with colitis also find complementary therapies such as yoga or acupuncture helpful.

Living with colitis can be tough, but there are ways to manage the condition and live a relatively normal life. With the right treatment, many people with colitis are able to control their symptoms and prevent flare-ups.

Can you suddenly develop colitis?

It's possible to suddenly develop colitis, although it's more common for the condition to develop gradually over time. Symptoms of colitis can include abdominal pain and cramping, bloody stool, diarrhea, fatigue, weight loss, and loss of appetite. If you experience any of these symptoms, it's important to see a doctor so that they can diagnose and treat the condition.

The exact cause of colitis is unknown, but it's thought to be the result of a combination of genetic and environmental factors. It's believed that colitis occurs when the body's immune system reacts abnormally to the bacteria in the digestive tract. This can cause inflammation and ulcers in the colon and rectum, which can lead to the symptoms of colitis.

There is no cure for colitis, but there are treatments that can help to control the symptoms and reduce the amount of inflammation in the digestive tract. Treatment options include medications, lifestyle changes, and surgery. Medications that are used to treat colitis include anti-inflammatory drugs, immune-suppressants, and antibiotics. Lifestyle changes that can help to manage symptoms include eating a healthy diet, avoiding foods that trigger symptoms, and getting enough rest. Surgery may be necessary in some cases to remove the diseased portion of the colon.

Living with colitis can be difficult, but there are ways to manage the condition and live a comfortable life. With the right treatment plan, many people with colitis are able to live normal, active lives.

Can colitis be cured with antibiotics?

There are many different types of colitis, each with their own unique set of causes, symptoms, and treatments. Some forms of colitis may be cured with antibiotics, while others may require other forms of treatment. It is important to speak with a medical professional to determine the best course of treatment for your particular case.

There are several different types of colitis, the most common being ulcerative colitis and Crohn's disease. Ulcerative colitis is a chronic inflammation of the lining of the colon and rectum. Crohn's disease is a chronic inflammatory disease of the gastrointestinal tract. Both of these conditions can be painful and may cause other problems such as diarrhea, weight loss, and fatigue.

While there is no cure for either ulcerative colitis or Crohn's disease, there are treatments available that can help to manage the symptoms and improve the quality of life for those affected. In some cases, antibiotics may be used to treat colitis. Antibiotics can help to clear the infection and reduce the inflammation. However, they are not effective for all types of colitis and may not be necessary in all cases.

Other treatments for colitis include immunosuppressants, biologics, and surgery. Immunosuppressants help to reduce the inflammation by suppressing the immune system. Biologics are a newer type of treatment that work by targeting specific parts of the immune system. Surgery is usually only considered when other treatments have failed.

If you are affected by colitis, it is important to speak with a medical professional to determine the best course of treatment for you. Depending on the type of colitis you have, there may be different treatment options available. Antibiotics may be an option for some, but not all, types of colitis. Other treatments, such as immunosuppressants, biologics, and surgery, may be necessary to manage the symptoms and improve the quality of life for those affected.

What is colitis pain like?

Colitis is a condition that affects the large intestine and causes inflammation and ulceration. The most common symptom of colitis is abdominal pain, often cramping pain that comes and goes. The pain may be mild or severe, and it may be constant or intermittent. Other symptoms of colitis may include diarrhea, constipation, blood in the stool, and weight loss.

Colitis pain can vary depending on the severity of the condition. For milder cases of colitis, the pain may be similar to that of other intestinal conditions, such as irritable bowel syndrome. The pain may be cramping and occur in waves, often after eating. More severe cases of colitis can cause intense pain that comes on suddenly and may be accompanied by nausea and vomiting. This type of pain may require hospitalization.

Is infectious colitis an autoimmune disease?

Infectious colitis is a condition that is characterized by inflammation of the large intestine, or colon. This condition can be caused by a variety of different infectious agents, including bacteria, viruses, and parasites. Infectious colitis is often associated with diarrhea, abdominal pain, and fever.

There is some debate as to whether or not infectious colitis is an autoimmune disease. Proponents of this theory point to the fact that infectious colitis is often associated with other autoimmune conditions, such as Crohn's disease and ulcerative colitis. Additionally, there is evidence to suggest that the inflammatory response in infectious colitis may be mediated by autoantibodies. However, further research is needed to confirm whether or not infectious colitis is truly an autoimmune disease.

It is important to note that infectious colitis is a serious condition that can lead to serious complications, such as dehydration and sepsis. If you suspect that you may have infectious colitis, it is important to seek medical attention immediately.

What happens if colitis is left untreated?

If colitis is left untreated, it can lead to a number of serious complications, including bleeding, dehydration, and malnutrition. Left untreated, colitis can also increase the risk of developing cancer of the colon. In addition, people with untreated colitis are at increased risk for developing other serious infections, such as Clostridium difficile (C. diff), a potentially life-threatening bacterial infection.

Colitis is a chronic inflammation of the inner lining of the colon and rectum. It is a debilitating disease that can lead to severe abdominal pain, bloody diarrhea, weight loss, and fatigue. There is no cure for colitis, but there are treatments available to help manage the symptoms and improve the quality of life for those affected by the disease.

What antibiotics treat infectious colitis?

Infectious colitis is a condition that is caused by an infection of the large intestine. The most common cause of infectious colitis is a bacterial infection, but it can also be caused by a virus or a parasite. Treatment for infectious colitis depends on the cause of the infection.

For bacterial infections, the most common cause of infectious colitis, antibiotics are the first line of treatment. The type of antibiotic used will depend on the specific bacteria that is causing the infection. Common antibiotics used to treat bacterial infections include ciprofloxacin, metronidazole, and amoxicillin.

Viral infections that cause infectious colitis are generally not treated with medication. The virus will usually go away on its own within a few days or weeks. However, there are some antiviral medications that can be used to treat viral colitis caused by the herpes simplex virus.

Parasitic infections that cause colitis are usually treated with antiparasitic medications. These medications kill the parasites that are causing the infection. Common antiparasitic medications used to treat colitis include metronidazole, albendazole, and nitazoxanide.

What is the difference between ulcerative colitis and infectious colitis?

Ulcerative colitis and infectious colitis are both disorders that affect the colon. The main difference between the two is that ulcerative colitis is a chronic condition while infectious colitis is acute.

Ulcerative colitis is characterized by inflammation and ulceration of the lining of the colon. This can lead to symptoms such as abdominal pain, diarrhea, and blood in the stool. Ulcerative colitis is usually a lifelong condition, although there may be periods of remission.

Infectious colitis is caused by an infection of the colon. This can be due to a virus, bacteria, or parasite. Infectious colitis typically only lasts for a short period of time and does not require long-term treatment. Symptoms of infectious colitis can include abdominal pain, diarrhea, and blood in the stool.

While ulcerative colitis and infectious colitis both affect the colon, there are some key differences between the two disorders. Ulcerative colitis is a chronic condition while infectious colitis is acute. In addition, ulcerative colitis is characterized by inflammation and ulceration of the colon while infectious colitis is caused by an infection of the colon.

Is colitis a stomach bug?

Colitis is not a stomach bug, but a condition of the large intestine. The large intestine, also known as the colon, is a long, coiled tube that removes water, electrolytes, and vitamins from indigestible food matter and stores the wastes that will eventually be eliminated from the body. The colon muscles propel the wastes through the intestines and into the rectum and anus, where they are eventually eliminated.

The large intestine is lined with a layer of mucus that protects it from the bacteria in the feces. The mucus also lubricates the movement of wastes through the intestine. In people with colitis, the colon mucus layer is inflamed and thickened. This inflammation can be caused by a number of things, including infection, irritation, and autoimmune reaction.

The symptoms of colitis vary depending on the severity of the inflammation, but can include abdominal pain, cramping, diarrhea, bloating, and weight loss. In some cases, the inflammation can be so severe that it leads to ulcers in the colon, bleeding, and perforation of the intestine.

Colitis is not a stomach bug, but a condition of the large intestine. The large intestine, also known as the colon, is a long, coiled tube that removes water, electrolytes, and vitamins from indigestible food matter and stores the wastes that will eventually be eliminated from the body. The colon muscles propel the wastes through the intestines and into the rectum and anus, where they are eventually eliminated.

The large intestine is lined with a layer of mucus that protects it from the bacteria in the feces. The mucus also lubricates the movement of wastes through the intestine. In people with colitis, the colon mucus layer is inflamed and thickened. This inflammation can be caused by a number of things, including infection, irritation, and autoimmune reaction.

The symptoms of colitis vary depending on the severity of the inflammation, but can include abdominal pain, cramping, diarrhea, bloating, and weight loss. In some cases, the inflammation can be so severe that it leads to ulcers in the colon, bleeding, and perforation of the intestine.

Can infectious colitis cause sepsis?

Infectious colitis is a condition that can occur when the large intestine becomes infected with bacteria, viruses, or parasites. Infectious colitis can cause a range of symptoms, from mild to severe, and in some cases, it can lead to sepsis.

Sepsis is a potentially life-threatening condition that occurs when an infection spreads throughout the body and triggers a widespread immune response. Infectious colitis can cause sepsis if the infection spreads beyond the large intestine and enters the bloodstream.

Infectious colitis is most commonly caused by bacterial infections, such as Salmonella, Shigella, E. coli, and Campylobacter. These bacteria are typically found in contaminated food or water, and they can cause severe diarrhea, abdominal pain, and fever.

Viral infections, such as norovirus and rotavirus, can also cause infectious colitis. These viruses are typically spread through contact with contaminated surfaces or food, and they can cause watery diarrhea, vomiting, and fever.

In some cases, parasitic infections can also lead to infectious colitis. The most common parasite that causes infectious colitis is Giardia lamblia. This parasite is found in contaminated food or water, and it can cause watery diarrhea, abdominal pain, and fatigue.

Infectious colitis can be a serious condition, and it can sometimes lead to sepsis. If you think you may have infectious colitis, it is important to see a doctor right away so that you can receive treatment and avoid complications.

Is Chicken OK for colitis?

When it comes to food and colitis, there is no one-size-fits-all answer. Some people with colitis can eat chicken without any problem, while others find that it exacerbates their symptoms.

If you have colitis, you may be wondering if chicken is a safe food to eat. There is no easy answer to this question, as everybody's experience with colitis is different. Some people find that chicken is fine to eat, while others find that it makes their colitis worse.

The best way to figure out if chicken is a trigger food for your colitis is to keep track of what you eat and how your body reacts. If you eat chicken and your colitis symptoms flare up, you may want to avoid chicken in the future. However, if you eat chicken and don't have any problems, it's probably safe for you to continue eating it.

If you're not sure whether chicken is a trigger food for your colitis, you may want to talk to a registered dietitian or your doctor. They can give you personalized advice about what to eat (or avoid) based on your individual situation.

Is colitis very painful?

Is colitis very painful? This is a question that needs to be answered on an individual basis, as the pain associated with colitis can vary greatly from person to person. However, it is generally agreed that colitis can be a very painful condition.

There are many different types of colitis, each with its own set of symptoms. However, pain is a common symptom among all types of colitis. The pain can be mild or severe, and it can come and go. It is often described as a sharp, cramping pain. Some people also experience pain in the rectum or anus.

The pain of colitis is often made worse by certain activities. For example, sitting for long periods of time can aggravate the pain, as can eating spicy or fatty foods. Some people find that their pain gets worse at night.

There are many different treatments for colitis, and the type of treatment will depend on the individual. Some people find that over-the-counter medications, such as ibuprofen, help to relieve their pain. Others may need to take prescription medications, such as steroids or immunosuppressants. Some people may need to have surgery to remove part of their colon.

No matter what treatment is used, it is important to remember that colitis is a serious condition and should not be ignored. If you are experiencing pain, it is important to speak to a doctor so that you can receive the treatment that you need.

Is colitis an emergency?

In short, colitis is not usually an emergency, but there are certain situations when it can be. If you have any concerns whatsoever, it is always best to consult with a medical professional.

If you are experiencing any sort of abdominal pain, cramping, bloating, or discomfort, along with rectal bleeding, sudden and persistent diarrhea, or vomiting, then you should seek medical attention right away. These could all be signs of a more serious condition, and it is always best to err on the side of caution.

If you have any sort of medical history that could predispose you to colitis, or if you have any other risk factors (such as being over the age of 50), then you should also speak to a doctor, even if you are not currently experiencing any symptoms. They will be able to advise you on the best course of action and help you to keep an eye on your condition.

Generally speaking, colitis is not an emergency, but there are certain situations when it can be. If you have any concerns whatsoever, it is always best to consult with a medical professional.

Colitis is a serious inflammation of the colon that can lead to a host of uncomfortable and even dangerous symptoms. While there is no cure for colitis, there are treatments available that can help to manage the symptoms and keep the condition under control. With the right treatment plan, many people with colitis are able to live relatively normal lives.

What is the best fruit for colitis?

There is no one definitive answer to this question as the best fruit for colitis may differ from person to person. Some people find that certain fruits trigger or worsen their symptoms, while others may tolerate them better. It is therefore important to experiment and find out what works best for you.

Some fruits that have been known to help with colitis include papaya, pineapple, and bananas. These fruits contain enzymes that may help to reduce inflammation in the gut. Other good options include green apples, apricots, and watermelon. These fruits are high in antioxidants and other nutrients that can help to support gut health.

It is generally advisable to avoid citrus fruits and berries, as these are more likely to cause irritation. However, as with all things, it is important to listen to your body and see what works for you. If you find that you can tolerate these fruits without any problems, then there is no reason to avoid them.

In general, it is best to eat fruits that are easy to digest and are not too acidic. This means that they are less likely to trigger symptoms or worsen existing inflammation. Experiment and see what works best for you – and always consult with your doctor if you are unsure about anything.

What to avoid during a colitis flare up?

When you're dealing with a colitis flare up, there are a few things you'll want to avoid. For one, you'll want to stay away from processed foods. This means no fast food, no prepackaged meals, and no processed snacks. You'll also want to avoid any food that could aggravate your symptoms, such as spicy food, dairy, and caffeine.

It's also important to avoid alcohol during a colitis flare up. Alcohol can irritate the lining of your gut, making your symptoms worse. If you're taking any medication for your colitis, you should also avoid drinking, as alcohol can interfere with the effectiveness of the medication.

Finally, you'll want to avoid anything that could stress you out. This means steering clear of stressful situations, getting enough sleep, and taking time to relax. When your body is under stress, it's more likely to experience a flare up.

By avoiding processed foods, spicy food, alcohol, and stress, you can help minimize the number and severity of your colitis flare ups.

Do you need a colonoscopy for colitis?

There is no simple answer to whether or not you need a colonoscopy for colitis. The reason for this is that there are many different types of colitis, and each type may require a different approach to treatment.

Some types of colitis, such as ulcerative colitis, are inflammatory diseases that can cause serious damage to the colon. In these cases, a colonoscopy may be necessary to assess the severity of the inflammation and to identify any ulcers or other damage. Other types of colitis, such as infectious colitis, are caused by infections and may not require a colonoscopy.

The decision about whether or not to have a colonoscopy for colitis will be made by your doctor based on the type of colitis you have, the severity of your symptoms, and any other factors that may be relevant. If you have any concerns about whether or not you need a colonoscopy, you should discuss them with your doctor.

What

color

is colitis poop?

When you have an inflammatory bowel disease like colitis, your poop can vary in color from day to day, depending on how inflamed your colon is. If your colon is only mildly inflamed, your poop might be close to its usual color. But if your colon is very inflamed, your poop might be red, yellow, or even green.

The color of your poop can also change depending on what you eat. If you eat a lot of green leafy vegetables, your poop might be green. If you eat beets, your poop might be red. And if you eat food that has a lot of artificial dyes in it, your poop might be any color of the rainbow!

But no matter what you eat, if you have colitis, your poop is likely to be softer than usual, and it might have a lot of mucus in it. (Mucus is that slimy stuff that helps keep your intestines lubricated.) You might also see blood in your stool, which can range from a few streaks of blood to large clots.

If you have any of these symptoms, it's important to see your doctor, because they could be signs of a serious bowel disease. But don't worry - with the right treatment, many people with colitis can lead happy, healthy lives.

When should you go to hospital with colitis?

If you have colitis, it is important to know when to go to the hospital. Some signs that you should go to the hospital are severe abdominal pain, rectal bleeding, weight loss, fevers, and constant nausea and vomiting. If you have any of these signs, you should contact your doctor immediately.

It is also important to know the signs of an impending flare-up. If you are having more than four bowel movements a day, your stools are watery or bloody, you are experiencing abdominal pain, or you are losing weight, you should contact your doctor. These may be signs that you are about to have a flare-up and should be seen by a doctor.

If you are having a flare-up, there are some things you can do at home to help manage your symptoms. Try to drink eight glasses of water a day, avoid high-fiber foods, and eat small, bland meals. You can also try over-the-counter medications like loperamide to help with diarrhea. However, if your symptoms are not improving or are getting worse, you should go to the hospital.

When you go to the hospital, the first thing the doctor will do is assess your symptoms. They will also likely order some tests, like a stool sample or blood tests. Once they have a diagnosis, they will be able to treat your colitis and help you manage your symptoms.

What is the main cause of ulcerative colitis?

Ulcerative colitis is caused by a combination of environmental and immunological factors. The main environmental factor is thought to be the hygiene hypothesis, which states that exposure to certain infectious agents early in life protects against the development of autoimmune diseases like ulcerative colitis. The main immunological factor is a defect in the mucosal immune system, which allows bacteria and other antigens to penetrate the mucosal barrier and trigger an inflammatory response.

What are the warning signs of ulcerative colitis?

There are a few warning signs that may indicate you have ulcerative colitis, a form of inflammatory bowel disease. If you have any of these symptoms, it's important to see a doctor to get a diagnosis:

Abdominal pain: This can range from a mild cramp to severe pain.

Diarrhea: This is a common symptom of ulcerative colitis. You may have watery stools or stools that contain blood.

Weight loss: This can happen because of the abdominal pain and diarrhea. You may also have a loss of appetite.

Fatigue: This can be caused by the inflammation in your body.

Fever: A fever may be present if you have inflammation in your body.

Rectal bleeding: This is a common symptom of ulcerative colitis. You may see blood on your toilet paper or in your stool.

Anemia: This can happen if you are losing blood from your gastrointestinal tract.

The causes of colitis can be many, from an infection to a more serious autoimmune condition. While the symptoms of colitis can be painful and debilitating, there are treatments available that can help. With the help of a doctor, people with colitis can find the right treatment for their individual case and learn to manage their condition.

Who is most likely to get ulcerative colitis?

Approximately 1 in 100 people in the United States have ulcerative colitis. The disease tends to run in families, so people with a first-degree relative (parent, child, or sibling) with ulcerative colitis have an increased risk of developing the disease. Ulcerative colitis also seems to be more common in people of Jewish descent.

Smoking cigarettes is a risk factor for developing ulcerative colitis, and people who smoke are less likely to respond to medical treatment for the disease.

People with ulcerative colitis are also at an increased risk of developing certain other conditions, including:

-Anemia

-Arthritis

-Skin problems

-Osteoporosis

-Liver disease

-Kidney stones

How do you make ulcerative colitis go away?

Ulcerative colitis is a chronic inflammation of the large intestine, also known as the colon. It is a form of inflammatory bowel disease (IBD), and can be incredibly painful, disruptive, and even life-threatening. The good news is that there are treatments available that can help to manage the symptoms and even make the disease go into remission.

The first step is to see a doctor or gastroenterologist to get a proper diagnosis. Once ulcerative colitis has been diagnosed, the next step is to develop a treatment plan. This will likely involve a combination of medication, lifestyle changes, and, in some cases, surgery.

Medications for ulcerative colitis can include anti-inflammatory drugs, immunosuppressants, and biologics. These can help to reduce inflammation and give some relief from symptoms. Lifestyle changes such as stress reduction, a healthy diet, and exercise can also help to manage symptoms and flares. In some cases, surgery may be necessary to remove part of the colon.

While there is no cure for ulcerative colitis, the goal of treatment is to make the disease go into remission. This means that there are no active symptoms and the inflammation has subsided. With proper treatment, many people with ulcerative colitis can lead normal, healthy lives.

Do you poop a lot with ulcerative colitis?

Ulcerative colitis (UC) is an inflammatory bowel disease (IBD). It causes inflammation and ulcers in the lining of your large intestine and rectum. The main symptom of active UC is bloody diarrhea. But UC can also cause other problems, like severe abdominal pain, fatigue, and weight loss.

People with UC often wonder how the disease will affect their bathroom habits. Some people worry that they will have to go to the bathroom more often, while others are concerned about having accidents.

There is no one answer to this question, as everyone experiences UC differently. Some people do have more frequent bowel movements, while others may have fewer. Some people find that their UC causes them to need to go to the bathroom more urgently, while others may not have this problem.

If you are concerned about how UC will affect your bathroom habits, it is best to talk to your doctor. They can offer advice and guidance based on your individual situation.

What is ulcerative colitis poop like?

The poop of someone with ulcerative colitis can vary in appearance, but typically it is watery, bloody, and mucus-filled. The Bristol Stool Scale is a seven-point scale that defines the different types of poop, and poop from someone with ulcerative colitis would typically be classified as type 6 or 7. This means that the poop is liquid, and often contains bits of undigested food or blood.

The appearance of ulcerative colitis poop can be alarming, but it is important to remember that it is not dangerous. The blood in the stool is usually from small lesions or ulcers in the colon, and does not indicate a serious medical condition. However, if you are experiencing other symptoms such as severe abdominal pain, fever, or weight loss, it is important to see a doctor.

Ulcerative colitis is a chronic inflammatory condition of the colon, and the poop symptoms are caused by the inflammation. The inflammation affects the ability of the colon to absorb water, which leads to the watery, loose stool. The inflammation can also cause ulcers and lesions in the colon, which can bleed and cause bloody stool. Additionally, the inflammation can cause mucus to be produced, which can also be seen in the stool.

Can you suddenly develop ulcerative colitis?

Ulcerative colitis (UC) is a chronic inflammatory bowel disease (IBD) that affects the mucosal layer of the large intestine, specifically the rectum and colon. Symptoms include bloody stool, abdominal pain, and weight loss. UC is believed to be caused by a combination of genetic and environmental factors.

There is no known cure for UC, but there are treatments available that can help to manage the symptoms and remission. UC is a lifelong condition, and it is important to be under the care of a doctor to help prevent any complications.

Can you suddenly develop ulcerative colitis?

There is no one answer to this question as everyone experiences UC differently. For some people, UC may develop gradually over time with no specific trigger, while for others, it may seem to come on suddenly. It is possible that a trigger (such as a virus or bacterial infection) may cause UC to flare up suddenly, but more research is needed to confirm this.

If you think you may have UC, it is important to see a doctor so that they can diagnose and treat the condition. Early diagnosis and treatment is important in reducing the severity of symptoms and preventing any long-term complications.

What foods heal colitis?

There is no one answer to the question of what foods heal colitis, as the condition can vary greatly from person to person. However, there are some general dietary guidelines that may help to ease the symptoms of colitis and promote healing.

Firstly, it is important to consume plenty of water and other fluids to prevent dehydration and keep the digestive system moving. Try to avoid caffeine and alcohol, as these can exacerbate dehydration and inflammation.

There are a few different types of colitis, and the specific diet recommendations may vary depending on the type. However, some general dietary guidelines for colitis include avoiding trigger foods, consuming smaller meals more frequently, and choosing nutrient-rich foods.

Trigger foods are different for everyone, but common triggers include spicy foods, greasy foods, and high-fiber foods. If a certain food seems to aggravate your colitis symptoms, it is best to avoid that food.

consuming smaller meals more frequently, and choosing nutrient-rich foods.

Nutrient-rich foods include plenty of fruits, vegetables, and whole grains. These foods contain important vitamins, minerals, and antioxidants that can help to reduce inflammation and promote healing. Omega-3 fatty acids are also beneficial for colitis, so including fish, nuts, and seeds in the diet is helpful. Probiotic-rich foods, such as yogurt and sauerkraut, are also beneficial for colitis sufferers as they help to promote a healthy balance of gut bacteria.

What should you not do if you have colitis?

If you have colitis, there are a few things you should avoid doing. First, you should not smoke. Smoking can make your colitis worse and can even lead to serious complications. Second, you should avoid drinking alcohol. Alcohol can also aggravate your colitis and can lead to dehydration. Third, you should avoid eating spicy or fatty foods. These types of foods can trigger a flare-up of your colitis. Finally, you should avoid stress. Stress can worsen your colitis symptoms and can even trigger a flare-up.

There is no easy answer when it comes to dealing with colitis. The best way to manage this condition is to work with a healthcare team to develop a plan that is right for you. There is no one-size-fits-all approach to managing colitis, so it is important to find an approach that works for you.

Does colitis get worse with age?

As we age, our bodies go through many changes. Unfortunately, some of these changes can lead to health problems, such as chronic diseases. One such chronic disease is colitis, which is a condition that affects the large intestine and causes inflammation.

There is no certain answer as to whether or not colitis gets worse with age. However, there are some risk factors that can increase the likelihood of the condition worsening. For example, older adults are more likely to have other chronic conditions that can make colitis worse, such as diabetes or heart disease. In addition, the immune system weakens with age, making it harder for the body to fight off inflammation.

If you have colitis, it is important to see your doctor regularly, even if you are not experiencing any symptoms. This is because colitis can flare up without warning and cause serious health complications. Treatment for colitis often includes medication, such as anti-inflammatory drugs, and making lifestyle changes, such as quitting smoking and eating a healthy diet.

If you are concerned about colitis getting worse as you age, talk to your doctor. They can help you manage your condition and minimize your risk of complications.

What happens if you ignore ulcerative colitis?

If you ignore ulcerative colitis, the condition will worsen and may lead to serious consequences. Without treatment, the inflammation will spread and damage the large intestine. This can lead to bleeding, pain, and diarrhea. In some cases, the inflammation can cause the large intestine to rupture. This is a life-threatening emergency that requires immediate medical attention. Ignoring ulcerative colitis can also lead to malnutrition and weight loss. This is because the inflammation makes it difficult for the body to absorb nutrients from food.

Left untreated, ulcerative colitis may also lead to colon cancer. This is a relatively rare complication, but it is more common in people with ulcerative colitis than in the general population. If you have ulcerative colitis, it is important to see a doctor and get treated. With proper treatment, most people with ulcerative colitis can live normal, healthy lives.

What are the stages of ulcerative colitis?

Ulcerative colitis is a chronic inflammatory disease of the colon. The most common symptom of ulcerative colitis is bloody diarrhea. Other symptoms may include abdominal pain, cramping, weight loss, and fatigue.

The course of ulcerative colitis varies from person to person. Some people have mild symptoms that come and go. Others have more severe symptoms that last for months or years. The symptoms may come and go in periods of remission and flare-up.

There are four stages of ulcerative colitis: mild, moderate, severe, and very severe.

Mild ulcerative colitis: Symptoms are present but not severe. There is bleeding from the rectum, but not enough to cause anemia. There is mild abdominal pain and cramping. weight loss is minimal.

Moderate ulcerative colitis: There is more frequent and severe bleeding from the rectum. Anemia is more common. There is moderate abdominal pain and cramping. weight loss is moderate.

Severe ulcerative colitis: There is continual bleeding from the rectum. Anemia is severe. There is severe abdominal pain and cramping. weight loss is severe.

Very severe ulcerative colitis: There is very severe bleeding from the rectum. Anemia is life-threatening. There is very severe abdominal pain and cramping. weight loss is extreme.

Ulcerative colitis is a chronic, relapsing-remitting disease. There is no cure for ulcerative colitis, but there are treatments that can help reduce the symptoms and improve the quality of life.

Can stress cause ulcerative colitis?

There is a lot of debate surrounding the topic of ulcerative colitis and stress. Some say that stress can be a trigger for ulcerative colitis, while others claim that there is no scientific evidence to support this theory. So, what is the truth?

It is difficult to say for certain whether or not stress can cause ulcerative colitis. This is because ulcerative colitis is a complex condition with many possible causes. However, some research suggests that stress may play a role in the development or worsening of ulcerative colitis.

For example, one study found that people with ulcerative colitis who reported higher levels of stress were more likely to experience a flare-up of their symptoms. Another study found that people with ulcerative colitis who had experienced a stressful life event were more likely to have a relapse of their symptoms.

So, while we cannot say for certain that stress causes ulcerative colitis, there is some evidence to suggest that it may be a contributing factor. If you are living with ulcerative colitis, it is important to manage your stress levels as best as you can. This may help to reduce the frequency and severity of your symptoms.

What foods soothe inflamed intestines?

When you have colitis, one of the last things you want to think about is food. You're probably feeling pretty crummy as it is, and the thought of eating anything probably doesn't sound all that appealing.

But the fact is, what you eat can make a big difference in how you feel. Some foods can help to soothe an inflamed intestine, while others can make the inflammation worse.

So

what should you eat if you have colitis?

Generally, a diet that is high in fiber and low in fat is best. This type of diet helps to bulk up the stool, which can make bowel movements easier and less painful.

Foods that are high in fiber include:

-Fruits, such as apples, bananas, and pears

-Vegetables, such as broccoli, carrots, and peas

-Whole-grain breads and cereals

-Beans

Another important part of a colitis diet is to make sure you're getting enough fluids. This helps to keep the stool soft and prevents constipation, which can be a real problem if you have colitis.

Good choices for fluids include:

-Water

-Juices

-Broth

-Decaffeinated tea

It's also important to avoid any foods that seem to make your symptoms worse. These "trigger" foods can vary from person to person, so you'll need to pay attention to your own body to figure out what to avoid. Some common trigger foods include:

-Dairy products

-Alcohol

-Caffeinated beverages

-Foods that are high in fat

-Spicy foods

-Raw fruits and vegetables

If you're not sure what trigger foods to avoid, you may want to talk to a registered dietitian. He or she can help you create a personalized diet plan that will meet your nutritional needs while also helping to keep your colitis symptoms under control.

What's the difference between colitis and ulcerative colitis?

Both colitis and ulcerative colitis are inflammatory bowel diseases (IBD). IBD is a condition that causes inflammation of the digestive tract. Colitis is a form of IBD that specifically refers to inflammation of the colon, while ulcerative colitis is a form of IBD that specifically refers to inflammation of the lining of the colon.

The main difference between colitis and ulcerative colitis is the location of the inflammation. Colitis refers to inflammation of the colon, while ulcerative colitis refers to inflammation of the lining of the colon. The symptoms of both diseases may be similar, but the severity of symptoms can vary depending on the location of the inflammation.

Colitis and ulcerative colitis are both serious conditions that can lead to a number of complications. If you think you may have either disease, it is important to see a doctor for a diagnosis.

Is ulcerative colitis serious?

Ulcerative colitis is a chronic inflammatory bowel disease that can be difficult to manage and, at times, may be serious. The exact cause of ulcerative colitis is unknown, but it is thought to be linked to an autoimmune reaction.

Symptoms of ulcerative colitis can vary, but may include abdominal pain, diarrhea, rectal bleeding, weight loss, and fatigue. Ulcerative colitis can also lead to complications, such as liver disease, osteoporosis, and an increased risk for colorectal cancer.

While there is no cure for ulcerative colitis, there are treatments available that can help to manage the symptoms and keep the disease under control. Treatment options include medication, surgery, and lifestyle changes.

Living with ulcerative colitis can be challenging, but it is important to keep in mind that the disease is not life-threatening. With proper treatment and self-care, many people with ulcerative colitis are able to live normal, active lives.

In conclusion, colitis is a serious condition that affects the colon. If left untreated, it can lead to life-threatening complications. Early diagnosis and treatment are essential to prevent the progression of the disease.

How do I know if I've got Crohn's?

There are a few different ways to find out whether or not you have Crohn's disease. The first step is to identify the symptoms. Symptoms of Crohn's disease can include: abdominal pain and cramping, diarrhea, weight loss, fatigue, fever, and bloody stools. If you experience any of these symptoms, it's important to see a doctor so they can rule out other potential causes.

In order to diagnose Crohn's disease, doctors will typically order a combination of blood tests, stool tests, and imaging tests. Blood tests can help to look for signs of inflammation, anemia, or infection. Stool tests can check for the presence of blood or pus in the stool, which can be indicative of Crohn's disease. Imaging tests, such as CT scans or MRIs, can be helpful in visualizing any inflammation or damage to the GI tract.

Once all of the test results are in, your doctor will be able to make a diagnosis of Crohn's disease. In some cases, a tissue biopsy may also be necessary in order to confirm the diagnosis. Crohn's disease is a chronic condition, which means that it is a lifelong condition that may flare up at times. Thankfully, there are a variety of treatments available that can help to manage the symptoms and keep the disease under control.

Can Crohn's disease go away?

Crohn's disease is a condition that causes inflammation of the digestive system. It is a chronic condition, which means it can last for a long time, and can go through periods of remission, where the symptoms get better, and then periods of flare-ups, when the symptoms get worse. There is no cure for Crohn's disease, but there are treatments that can help to manage the symptoms and keep the condition under control.

The main symptom of Crohn's disease is abdominal pain, and other symptoms can include diarrhoea, weight loss, and fatigue. Crohn's disease can also affect other parts of the body, such as the skin, eyes, and joints.

In some people, Crohn's disease can go away on its own, but it is more likely to be a long-term condition. Even if the symptoms go away, the underlying inflammation can still be present, and the condition can flare up again at any time.

Most people with Crohn's disease will need to take medication to manage the symptoms, and some people may need to have surgery to remove the affected parts of the digestive system.

What do Crohn's pains feel like?

When flare-ups of Crohn's disease occur, they can cause a great deal of pain. The pain may be diffuse, felt all over the abdomen, or it may be localized to a specific area. The pain may be crampy, like menstrual cramps, or it may be sharp and stabbing. Typically, the pain comes in waves, with periods of no pain in between.

Crohn's disease can also cause pain in the joints and muscles, as well as headaches and mouth sores. The pain from Crohn's disease can be debilitating, making it hard to get up and about, and to participate in normal activities. The pain may also be severe enough to interfere with sleep.

There are a number of treatments available to help manage the pain of Crohn's disease. Medications, both over-the-counter and prescription, can be helpful in reducing the pain. In some cases, surgery may be necessary to remove the diseased portion of the intestine.

If you are experiencing pain due to Crohn's disease, it is important to talk to your doctor. They can help you to determine the best course of treatment for your individual situation.

What will happen if Crohn's disease is left untreated?

Crohn's disease is an inflammatory bowel disease (IBD) that can cause severe abdominal pain, fatigue, weight loss, and diarrhea. If left untreated, Crohn's disease can lead to life-threatening complications such as intestinal blockages, fistulas, and malnutrition. In severe cases, Crohn's disease can also cause death.

What can trigger Crohn's disease?

There are a variety of things that can trigger Crohn's disease. Some triggers may be more common than others, and some people may be more susceptible to certain triggers than others.

Dietary triggers are thought to be one of the most common, with certain foods and drinks potentially causing inflammation in the gut. Foods that are high in fat and sugar are thought to be particularly problematic, as well as dairy products, gluten, and spicy or acidic foods. Some people also find that they have a sensitivity to nightshade vegetables like tomatoes, potatoes, and peppers.

Infections are another potential trigger for Crohn's disease. Both bacterial and viral infections have been linked to the development of the condition, and it's thought that the gut bacteria may play a particularly important role. People who have had a history of gut infections are thought to be at an increased risk of developing Crohn's disease.

Certain medications have also been linked to Crohn's disease, particularly non-steroidal anti-inflammatory drugs (NSAIDs) and antibiotics. It's thought that these medications can disrupt the delicate balance of gut bacteria, which may lead to inflammation.

Finally, stress has been identified as a potential trigger for Crohn's disease. It's thought that stress can worsen the symptoms of the condition and may even play a role in its development.

Can you drink alcohol with Crohn's disease?

It's a common question for people with Crohn's disease: can you drink alcohol? There is no easy yes or no answer, as it depends on a number of factors.

First, it's important to know that alcohol can worsen the symptoms of Crohn's disease. It's a

inflammatory disease, and alcohol is a known inflammatory. This means that drinking alcohol can make the symptoms of Crohn's disease, such as abdominal pain and diarrhea, worse.

Second, it's important to consider how alcohol will interact with the medications you're taking for Crohn's disease. Some medications, such as methotrexate, can be made less effective by alcohol. Others, such as prednisone, can make you more susceptible to the side effects of alcohol, such as liver damage.

Finally, it's important to be honest with yourself about how well you can handle alcohol. Crohn's disease can be unpredictable, and you may not be able to drink as much as you used to. It's important to be mindful of how alcohol will affect you both physically and mentally.

If you do decide to drink, it's important to do so in moderation. One or two drinks a day is generally considered to be safe for people with Crohn's disease. But, as always, it's important to listen to your body and drink only what feels comfortable for you.

What age does

Crohns

start?

Crohn's disease can affect people of all ages, but it's most commonly diagnosed in people in their twenties and thirties. The disease can be difficult to diagnose because its symptoms, like abdominal pain and diarrhea, are similar to other gastrointestinal conditions.

There are a few risk factors that may increase your chances of developing Crohn's disease, including:

* Having a family member with the disease

* Smoking

* Having another inflammatory bowel disease, like ulcerative colitis

If you have Crohn's disease, you may experience a range of symptoms that can range from mild to severe. Common symptoms include:

* Abdominal pain and cramping

* Diarrhea

* Rectal bleeding

* Weight loss

* Fatigue

Crohn's disease can also cause other problems outside of the digestive system. For example, you may have skin rashes, joint pain, and eye inflammation.

While there is no cure for Crohn's disease, there are treatments that can help manage the symptoms and improve your quality of life. Treatment options include:

* Medications: There are a number of different medications that can be used to treat Crohn's disease. These include anti-inflammatory drugs, immune-system suppressors, and antibiotics.

* Surgery: In some cases, surgery may be needed to remove the diseased part of the intestine.

* Dietary changes: Eating a healthy diet and avoiding trigger foods can help manage symptoms.

If you think you may have Crohn's disease, it's important to see a doctor so that you can get an accurate diagnosis and start treatment.

There is currently no cure for colitis, however with proper management and treatment, symptoms can be greatly reduced and remission can be achieved. It is important to see a doctor if you think you may have colitis, as leaving it untreated can lead to serious complications. With the right treatment plan, people with colitis can lead happy and healthy lives.

What worsens Crohn's disease?

There is no one definitive answer to this question as Crohn's disease is a complex condition with many possible contributing factors. However, there are some common triggers that can make symptoms worse. These include stress, smoking, eating certain foods, and taking certain medications.

Stress is a significant factor in many chronic illnesses, and Crohn's disease is no exception. Stress can contribute to flare-ups and make symptoms worse. Try to find healthy ways to manage stress, such as exercise, journaling, or spending time with friends and family.

Smoking is also a trigger for Crohn's disease. If you smoke, quitting is one of the best things you can do for your health. Talk to your doctor about quitting smoking and they can help you find resources to make it easier.

Certain foods can also trigger Crohn's disease symptoms. These vary from person to person, but common triggers include spicy foods, dairy products, and foods high in fat. Keeping a food diary can help you identify which foods make your symptoms worse.

Finally, certain medications can also trigger Crohn's disease symptoms. Non-steroidal anti-inflammatory drugs (NSAIDs), for example, are a common trigger. If you take NSAIDs for another condition, speak to your doctor about alternatives.

What foods heal Crohn's disease?

There is no one-size-fits-all answer to the question of what foods heal Crohn's disease, as each individual's body and condition is unique. However, there are certain foods that are known to be beneficial for Crohn's sufferers, and it is generally recommended to consume a diet that is high in fiber and low in fat.

Some of the best foods for Crohn's disease are those that are rich in fiber, as this helps to bulk up stools and ease constipation (a common symptom of Crohn's). Good sources of fiber include fruits, vegetables, whole grains, and legumes. It is also important to stay hydrated, so make sure to drink plenty of water throughout the day.

Another crucial element of a Crohn's-friendly diet is avoiding trigger foods. These are different for everyone, but common trigger foods include dairy, caffeine, alcohol, and spicy or fatty foods. If you are unsure which foods trigger your Crohn's symptoms, it may be helpful to keep a food diary and note when you experience flares.

While there is no cure for Crohn's disease, making dietary changes can often help to ease symptoms and improve overall quality of life. Simply speaking with a registered dietitian can be a great first step in finding the right Crohn's-friendly diet for you.

Can I live a normal life with

Crohns

?

Many people with Crohn's disease can lead normal, active lives. Some people have Crohn's disease that is very mild, with few or no symptoms.

Other people have Crohn's disease that is more severe, with more frequent and intense symptoms.

Most people with Crohn's disease will have periods of time when they feel well and their symptoms are not present, intermingled with periods of time when they have an active disease and do experience symptoms. Even people with more severe Crohn's disease can have long periods of remission, when they feel well and have no or very few symptoms.

There are a number of different treatments available that can help people with Crohn's disease manage their symptoms and achieve remission. Some people with Crohn's disease will need to take medication on a long-term basis, while others may only need medication during active periods of disease.

People with Crohn's disease can also make lifestyle changes that can help to manage their symptoms and improve their quality of life. These changes can include eating a healthy diet, getting regular exercise, and avoiding smoking.

Crohn's disease is a chronic condition, which means that it is a long-term condition that cannot be cured. However, with treatment, many people with Crohn's disease can lead normal, active lives.

What is Crohn's disease NZ?

Crohn's disease is an inflammatory bowel disease (IBD) that primarily affects the small intestine. The major symptoms of Crohn's disease include abdominal pain, diarrhea, and weight loss. Crohn's disease can also lead to intestinal bleeding, intestinal obstruction, and perforation of the intestine.

Crohn's disease is a chronic, relapsing condition that is characterized by periods of remission (when symptoms are not present) interspersed with flare-ups (when symptoms reappear). The severity of Crohn's disease varies from person to person and can range from mild to life-threatening. There is currently no cure for Crohn's disease, but treatment can help to control symptoms and improve quality of life.

Crohn's disease is a type of IBD that specifically affects the small intestine. However, Crohn's disease can also affect other parts of the digestive system, including the mouth, esophagus, stomach, and large intestine. Crohn's disease is an autoimmune disease, which means that it occurs when the body's immune system mistakenly attacks healthy tissue. The exact cause of Crohn's disease is unknown, but it is thought to be due to a combination of genetic and environmental factors.

Crohn's disease is more common in developed countries, such as New Zealand, and it is estimated that 1 in every 1,000 people in New Zealand has the condition. Crohn's disease can affect people of any age, but it is most commonly diagnosed in young adults between the ages of 15 and 30. Crohn's disease is more common in people of Caucasian descent, and it is slightly more common in women than in men.

Can you develop Crohn's late in life?

It's not uncommon for Crohn's disease to develop later in life. While the average age of diagnosis is between 20 and 30 years old, it's not unheard of for people to be diagnosed in their 50s or 60s.

There are a variety of factors that can contribute to the development of Crohn's disease later in life. One possibility is that the disease progresses more slowly in older people, which can make it harder to diagnose. Another possibility is that people are more likely to have atypical symptoms as they age, which can make the disease harder to identify.

It's important to remember that Crohn's disease can affect people of any age, and that early diagnosis and treatment is essential for managing the disease. If you have any concerns about your health, it's important to speak to your doctor.

Does Crohn's show up in a blood test?

Blood tests can be useful in diagnosing Crohn's disease, but they are not always definitive. In some cases, Crohn's disease may not show up on a blood test at all. In other cases, the test may show evidence of inflammation, but it may not be clear if the inflammation is due to Crohn's disease or another condition. In some cases, a blood test may show evidence of Crohn's disease, but further testing will be needed to confirm the diagnosis.

Can I test for Crohn's at home?

Crohn's disease is a form of inflammatory bowel disease (IBD). It is a chronic condition that can cause severe symptoms and can be very debilitating. There is no cure for Crohn's disease, but there are treatments that can help to manage the symptoms and improve the quality of life for those who have the condition.

One of the most important aspects of managing Crohn's disease is early diagnosis. If the condition is diagnosed early, it is possible to treat it more effectively and prevent serious complications from developing.

There are a number of tests that can be used to diagnose Crohn's disease, but they can be expensive and invasive. Many people with Crohn's disease are keen to find a way to test for the condition at home, without having to go through the hassle and expense of seeing a doctor.

There are a number of home test kits available that claim to be able to diagnose Crohn's disease. However, it is important to be aware that these tests are not always accurate. Some of them are based on outdated information, and none of them are as reliable as a diagnosis made by a qualified medical professional.

If you are worried that you may have Crohn's disease, the best thing to do is to see your doctor. They will be able to carry out the necessary tests and give you a definitive diagnosis.

There is no one-size-fits-all answer to the question of how to treat colitis, as the condition varies greatly from person to person. However, some general tips on managing the condition include eating a healthy diet, avoiding trigger foods, and managing stress levels. In some cases, medication may also be necessary to control inflammation and symptoms. With proper treatment, many people with colitis are able to lead normal, healthy lives.

Can you heal Crohn's with diet?

There's no surefire Crohn's disease diet. But some foods may make symptoms worse, while others might help you feel better. The key is to experiment to see what works for you.

Crohn's disease is an inflammatory bowel disorder that can lead to abdominal pain, severe diarrhea, fatigue, weight loss and malnutrition. There is no cure for Crohn's, but there are treatments that can help manage the symptoms.

Diet is often thought of as a natural way to treat Crohn's disease. And there's some evidence that certain foods may help ease symptoms.

The specific carbohydrate diet (SCD) is a popular diet for Crohn's disease. The diet is based on the theory that Crohn's is caused by an overgrowth of bacteria in the intestines. The SCD eliminates most carbohydrates, which the theory suggests will starve the bacteria and help heal the intestines.

There's some evidence that the SCD may help ease Crohn's symptoms. A small study published in the Journal of Clinical Gastroenterology found that the SCD helped improve symptoms in children with Crohn's disease.

However, the SCD is a very restrictive diet, and it can be hard to stick to. There's also no evidence that the diet is effective in the long term.

Other elimination diets, such as the gluten-free diet, the low-FODMAP diet and the paleo diet, have also been studied for their potential to ease Crohn's symptoms.

There's some evidence that a gluten-free diet may help Crohn's symptoms. A study published in the American Journal of Gastroenterology found that a gluten-free diet helped improve symptoms in people with Crohn's disease who did not have celiac disease.

The low-FODMAP diet is a diet that eliminates certain short-chain carbohydrates that are thought to contribute to gastrointestinal distress. The diet has been shown to be effective in easing the symptoms of irritable bowel syndrome (IBS), and there's some evidence that it may also help Crohn's symptoms.

A study published in the Journal of Clinical Gastroenterology found that the low-FODMAP diet helped improve symptoms in people with Crohn's disease.

The paleo diet is a way of eating that mimics the way our hunter-gatherer ancestors ate. The diet is based on the premise that modern diseases are caused by the Western diet, which is high in processed foods, refined carbs and sugar.

The paleo diet has been shown to improve the symptoms of inflammatory disorders like Crohn's disease. A study published in the Journal of Clinical Gastroenterology found that the paleo diet helped improve symptoms in people with Crohn's disease.

Is Crohn's disease Painful?

Is Crohn's disease painful? While the symptoms of Crohn's disease can vary from person to person, the majority of those affected by the condition do experience pain. The pain associated with Crohn's disease is typically a result of inflammation in the digestive tract. This inflammation can cause a wide variety of symptoms, including abdominal pain, diarrhea, and weight loss. In some cases, the pain may be so severe that it leads to hospitalization. While there is no cure for Crohn's disease, there are treatments available that can help to control the symptoms and lessen the pain.

What is the difference between Crohn's and IBS?

There are two main types of colitis, Crohn's colitis and ulcerative colitis. Both involve inflammation of the large intestine, but there are some key differences between the two.

Crohn's colitis is a type of inflammatory bowel disease (IBD). It can affect any part of the gastrointestinal tract from the mouth to the anus, but most commonly affects the small intestine. Crohn's colitis is characterized by deep ulcerations and inflammation in the lining of the intestine.

Ulcerative colitis, on the other hand, is a chronic inflammatory condition that only affects the large intestine or colon. The inflammation in ulcerative colitis is limited to the innermost lining of the colon and typically only affects the lower part of the intestine.

There are several key differences between Crohn's and ulcerative colitis. Crohn's colitis is more likely to be associated with fever, weight loss, and fatigue. It can also cause anal fissures and fistulas (abnormal connections between tissues). Ulcerative colitis is more likely to cause bloody stool and abdominal pain. Additionally, people with ulcerative colitis are at an increased risk for developing colon cancer.

While there is no cure for either Crohn's colitis or ulcerative colitis, both can be managed with medication and lifestyle changes. Crohn's colitis is typically treated with a combination of anti-inflammatory drugs and immune-suppressants. Ulcerative colitis is usually treated with anti-inflammatory drugs, immune-suppressants, and/or 5-aminosalicylates. Surgery may also be an option for people with Crohn's colitis or ulcerative colitis who do not respond to medication.

While Crohn's colitis and ulcerative colitis share some similarities, there are also some key differences between the two types of colitis. It is important to be aware of these differences so that you can get the most appropriate treatment for your condition.

Can food cause Crohn's flare?

It is not known what causes Crohn's disease, but there are many theories. One theory is that a viral or bacterial infection can trigger the disease. Another theory is that Crohn's is caused by an overreaction of the immune system. There is also evidence that Crohn's may be caused by a combination of genetic and environmental factors.

There is no definitive answer to the question of whether or not food can cause Crohn's flare. However, there are some things that may trigger a flare-up. These triggers may be different for different people. Some common triggers include:

- Dairy products
- fatty foods
- foods high in fiber
- spicy foods
- alcohol
- tobacco

If you have Crohn's disease, it is important to pay attention to your body and what triggers your flares. You may want to keep a food diary to help you identify your triggers. You should also work with a registered dietitian to ensure that you are getting the nutrients you need.

Do you need medication for Crohn's?

There is no one-size-fits-all answer to this question – the decision of whether or not to take medication for Crohn's disease will be unique to each individual. Some people with Crohn's disease will find that their symptoms can be controlled through lifestyle changes and diet, and medication may not be necessary. Others may find that their symptoms are more severe, or do not respond to lifestyle changes, and will require medication to keep them under control.

There are a range of different medication options available for Crohn's disease, and the decision of which to take (if any) will be based on a number of factors, including the severity of symptoms, the person's age and health, other medications they are taking, and any potential side-effects.

Some of the most common medication options for Crohn's disease include:

Anti-inflammatory drugs: These can help to reduce inflammation in the gut, and are often the first line of treatment for Crohn's disease.

Immunomodulators: These work by modulating the immune system, and can be effective in people who do not respond to anti-inflammatory drugs.

Biologics: These are a newer type of medication, and work by targeting specific parts of the immune system. They are usually only considered for people who have not responded to other treatments.

Surgery is also an option for some people with Crohn's disease, and may be recommended if medication is not effective in controlling symptoms, or if there are complicating factors such as a blockage in the gut.

Making the decision of whether or not to take medication for Crohn's disease is a personal one, and should be made in consultation with a healthcare professional. They will be able to advise on the best course of treatment based on the individual's specific circumstances.

Where does Crohn's pain start?

Pain from Crohn's disease can originate from many different places in the gastrointestinal tract. The most common location is the last portion of the small intestine, called the ileum, where approximately 70% of people with Crohn's disease experience pain. The pain is usually a dull, cramping sensation that comes and goes. It is often worse after eating, and can wake people up at night.

Other potential sources of Crohn's pain include inflammation of the stomach and the first part of the small intestine, called the duodenum. Inflammation of the large intestine, or colon, is also a frequent cause of pain. In addition, people with Crohn's disease may experience pain in other parts of their body, including their joints, skin, and eyes. This is because Crohn's disease is an inflammatory condition, and inflammation can occur in any part of the body.

Crohn's disease is a chronic condition, which means that the pain associated with it can be long-lasting. Although there are treatments that can help to reduce the pain, it is not always possible to completely eliminate it. For some people, the pain from Crohn's disease can be mild and only occasional, while for others it can be severe and constant. No matter how severe the pain is, it can be a very debilitating and frustrating symptom of Crohn's disease.

How do doctors test for Crohn's?

There is no single test for Crohn's disease. Rather, doctors use a combination of tests to make a diagnosis.

The first step is usually a physical exam. Your doctor will ask about your symptoms and medical history. They will also check for signs of Crohn's, such as abdominal pain, weight loss, and diarrhea.

Your doctor may also order blood tests. These can help check for anemia or inflammation. They can also rule out other conditions that may cause similar symptoms, such as celiac disease.

Imaging tests may also be ordered. These can help show changes in the intestines that are characteristic of Crohn's. Common imaging tests include X-rays, computed tomography (CT) scans, and magnetic resonance imaging (MRI) scans.

The final step in diagnosing Crohn's is usually a colonoscopy or upper endoscopy. During these procedures, a thin, flexible tube is inserted into the rectum or upper digestive tract. The tube has a light and a camera, which allows the doctor to get a close look at the intestines. Biopsies can also be taken during these procedures. A biopsy is a small piece of tissue that is removed and examined under a microscope.

There is no single test that can definitively diagnose Crohn's disease. However, a combination of tests can help your doctor make a diagnosis.

There is no one-size-fits-all approach to managing colitis, but there are many ways to manage the condition and keep it under control. Some people may need medication to control their symptoms, while others may be able to manage their colitis with diet and lifestyle changes. The important thing is to work with your doctor to find the approach that works best for you.

What is Crohn's disease symptoms in females?

Crohn's disease is an inflammatory bowel disease that can affect any part of the digestive tract, from the mouth to the anus. The main symptoms of Crohn's disease are abdominal pain and diarrhea, although other symptoms can include weight loss, fatigue, and fever.

Crohn's disease is more common in women than in men, and the symptoms can vary depending on the location and severity of the inflammation. The most common symptom of Crohn's disease in women is abdominal pain, which is often severe and may be accompanied by diarrhea. Other common symptoms include weight loss, fatigue, and fever.

In some cases, Crohn's disease can also cause complications such as fistulas (abnormal connections between different parts of the body), abscesses (collections of pus), and malnutrition. Crohn's disease is a chronic condition, which means that it can last for many years and may flare up or go into remission at different times. There is no cure for Crohn's disease, but there are treatments that can help to control the symptoms and minimize the risk of complications.

What can cause ischemic colitis?

Ischemic colitis (IC) is a condition in which the blood supply to the large intestine becomes blocked. This can happen due to a number of different reasons, including:

-Narrowing of the arteries that supply blood to the large intestine

-A tear in the lining of the intestine

-An inflammation of the blood vessels

-A blockage in the lymphatic system

IC is more common in older adults, and it is estimated that it affects around 1 in every 1,000 people over the age of 60. There are a number of different factors that can increase your risk of developing IC, including:

-A history of smoking

-A history of heart disease

-A history of Crohn's disease or ulcerative colitis

-A history of blood clots

If you have any of these risk factors, it's important to talk to your doctor about how to best reduce your risk of developing IC.

IC can often be difficult to diagnose, as the symptoms can be similar to other conditions, such as Crohn's disease or irritable bowel syndrome. However, there are a few key symptoms that are more likely to be associated with IC, including:

-Abdominal pain that is typically relieved by passing stool

-Blood in the stool

-Diarrhea

-Nausea and vomiting

If you experience any of these symptoms, it's important to see your doctor so that they can rule out other potential causes and properly diagnose your condition.

There is no one-size-fits-all treatment for IC, as the best approach depends on the underlying cause of the condition. However, some common treatments include:

-Medications to improve blood flow to the intestine

-Surgery to remove a blockage in the intestine

-Antibiotics to clear an infection

In most cases, IC can be successfully treated with one of these approaches. However, in some cases, IC may lead to more serious complications, such as:

-Anemia

-Bowel obstruction

-Kidney failure

-Perforation of the intestine

If you have IC, it's important to see your doctor regularly so that they can monitor your condition and make sure that it's being properly treated. If you develop any new or worsening symptoms, it's also important to see your doctor right away so that they can assess whether or not your condition is worsening.

How do you fix ischemic colitis?

Ischemic colitis occurs when there is insufficient blood flow to the large intestine. This can happen as a result of a blockage in the arteries that supply blood to the intestine, or it can be a result of a low level of oxygen in the blood. Treatment for ischemic colitis involves restoring blood flow to the intestine. This can be done through surgery, angioplasty, or thrombolytic therapy. Surgery is the most common treatment for ischemic colitis. During surgery, the surgeon will make an incision in the abdomen and remove the blockage from the artery. Angioplasty is a less invasive alternative to surgery. During angioplasty, a small balloon is inserted into the blocked artery and inflated. This opens up the artery and restores blood flow to the intestine. Thrombolytic therapy is a less common treatment for ischemic colitis. During thrombolytic therapy, a medication is injected into the blocked artery. The medication dissolves the blood clot and restores blood flow to the intestine.

What is the difference between colitis and ischemic colitis?

There are many different types of colitis, but the two most common types are colitis and ischemic colitis. Colitis is an inflammation of the colon, while ischemic colitis is a lack of blood flow to the colon. Both conditions can cause severe abdominal pain, diarrhea, and bleeding.

Colitis is often caused by infection, inflammation, or autoimmune diseases. Infectious colitis is usually caused by bacteria, viruses, or parasites. Inflammatory colitis is often caused by Crohn's disease or ulcerative colitis.

Autoimmune colitis is often caused by autoimmune conditions such as celiac disease.

Ischemic colitis is often caused by a blockage in the arteries that supply blood to the colon. This blockage can be caused by atherosclerosis, thrombosis, or embolism. Ischemic colitis can also be caused by medications that constrict blood vessels, such as nonsteroidal anti-inflammatory drugs (NSAIDs).

The symptoms of colitis and ischemic colitis are similar, but there are some key differences. Colitis often causes bloody diarrhea, while ischemic colitis typically does not. Ischemic colitis is also more likely to cause fever, nausea, and vomiting.

The treatment for colitis and ischemic colitis is also similar, but there are some key differences. Colitis is often treated with antibiotics, anti-inflammatory drugs, or immune-suppressive drugs. Ischemic colitis is often treated with surgery to remove the blockage in the arteries supplying blood to the colon.

What foods should I avoid with ischemic colitis?

Ischemic colitis is a condition that occurs when blood flow to the colon is reduced. This can cause the colon to become inflamed and may lead to some uncomfortable symptoms.

There are a few things you can do to help manage your condition and one of them is paying attention to the foods you eat. While there is no specific diet for ischemic colitis, there are certain foods that can trigger symptoms or make them worse.

Some of the foods you may want to avoid include:

- spicy foods

- high-fat foods

- fried foods

- processed foods

- dairy products

- caffeine

- alcohol

Of course, everyone is different and you may find that you can tolerate some of these foods better than others. It is important to experiment a little and find out what works best for you. You may also want to talk to a registered dietitian who can help you create a nutritious and well-balanced diet that meets your specific needs.

Is ischemic colitis fatal?

Ischemic colitis is a condition that occurs when blood flow to the colon is decreased. This can happen due to a blockage in the blood vessels or a decrease in the production of blood. When blood flow is decreased, the cells in the colon begin to die. This can lead to inflammation and ulcers in the colon.

Ischemic colitis can be a very serious condition, and it can be fatal in some cases. If the blood flow to the colon is not restored, the cells in the colon will continue to die. This can cause the colon to rupture, and the contents of the colon will leak into the abdomen. This can lead to a serious infection, and it can be fatal.

Ischemic colitis is a medical emergency, and it should be treated as such. If you think you may have ischemic colitis, you should go to the hospital immediately.

How long does it take for a bowel to become ischemic?

The colon, or large intestine, is a muscular tube about five feet long that connects the small intestine to the rectum and anus. The main function of the colon is to absorb water and electrolytes from indigestible food matter and to store waste matter until it is eliminated.

The large intestine has three main sections: the ascending colon, the transverse colon, and the descending colon. The ascending colon starts at the cecum, the blind sac at the end of the small intestine, and runs up the right side of the abdomen. The transverse colon crosses the abdomen from right to left. The descending colon starts at the splenic flexure, where the descending colon meets the transverse colon, and runs down the left side of the abdomen. The sigmoid colon is the S-shaped section of the descending colon that connects to the rectum.

The colon is supplied by blood vessels that run along its surface and by a network of nerves. The blood supply to the colon comes from the inferior mesenteric artery, which branches off of the aorta. The inferior mesenteric artery supplies blood to the descending and sigmoid colon. The blood vessels that run along the surface of the colon are called the vasa recta.

The colon is innervated by the sympathetic and parasympathetic nervous systems. The sympathetic nervous system is responsible for the "fight-or-flight" response and increases heart rate and blood pressure. The parasympathetic nervous system is responsible for the "rest and digest" response and slows heart rate and decreases blood pressure.

The colon is a very important part of the digestive system and plays a vital role in absorption and elimination. The colon is a site of many different diseases and disorders, including colitis.

Colitis is a condition that results in inflammation of the colon. The inflammation can be caused by a number of different things, including infection, irritation, or autoimmune diseases. Colitis can be a very mild condition that causes a few intestinal issues, or it can be a severe, life-threatening condition.

The symptoms of colitis depend on the severity of the inflammation. Mild symptoms may include abdominal pain, diarrhea, and blood in the stool. More severe symptoms may include severe abdominal pain, fever, weight loss, and dehydration.

Colitis is treated depending on the cause of the inflammation. If the inflammation is caused by an infection, the treatment may include antibiotics. If the inflammation is caused by irritants, the treatment may include surface-active agents. If the inflammation is caused by an autoimmune disease, the treatment may include immunosuppressive drugs.

The prognosis of colitis depends on the severity of the condition. Mild colitis may go away on its own, or it may require treatment to resolve. More severe colitis may require hospitalization and may be life-threatening.

Colitis is a serious inflammation of the colon that can have many causes. While some forms of colitis are temporary and treatable, others can be chronic and life-threatening. Early diagnosis and treatment is essential to preventing serious complications.

Can a colonoscopy detect ischemic colitis?

A colonoscopy is a diagnostic procedure that is used to evaluate the large intestine for possible causes of symptoms such as bleeding, abdominal pain, changes in bowel habits, or weight loss. The colonoscopy may also be used as a screening test for colorectal cancer. The colonoscope is a long, narrow, flexible tube that is equipped with a light and a camera. The camera allows the doctor to see the inside of the colon.

During the colonoscopy, the doctor may take biopsies (samples of tissue) to be sent to the laboratory for further testing. Ischemic colitis is a condition that occurs when there is not enough blood flow to the large intestine. This can cause the tissues of the intestine to become inflamed and ulcerated. Ischemic colitis can be caused by a variety of conditions, including atherosclerosis, thrombosis, vasculitis, and medications.

The symptoms of ischemic colitis include abdominal pain, bloody stools, and diarrhea. Ischemic colitis is a potentially serious condition that can lead to serious complications such as colon perforation, sepsis, and death. prompt diagnosis and treatment are essential.

A colonoscopy is the best diagnostic tool for ischemic colitis. The colonoscope can be used to visualise the inflamed and ulcerated tissue. The biopsies taken during the colonoscopy can be used to confirm the diagnosis. Ischemic colitis is a potentially serious condition that requires prompt diagnosis and treatment.

Can I drink coffee with ischemic colitis?

Inflammatory bowel disease (IBD), such as ulcerative colitis and Crohn's disease, can cause gastrointestinal symptoms like abdominal pain, diarrhea, and weight loss. Coffee is a common trigger for IBD symptoms, so many people with IBD avoid drinking coffee. However, coffee may not be the only trigger for IBD symptoms. Some people with IBD can drink coffee without experiencing any symptoms.

There is no one-size-fits-all answer to whether or not you can drink coffee with IBD. Some people find that they can drink coffee without any issues. Others find that coffee makes their symptoms worse. If you have IBD, you will need to experiment to see what works for you.

If you have IBD and you want to drink coffee, there are a few things you can do to minimize your risk of triggering symptoms. First, avoid coffee that is very acidic. Start with a milder coffee, such as a light roast, and see how your body reacts. You may also want to try brewing your coffee with less water to make it stronger. If you have trouble drinking coffee without triggering symptoms, you may want to try decaffeinated coffee or caffeine-free alternatives.

It's important to remember that everyone is different. What works for one person with IBD may not work for another. If you have IBD and you want to drink coffee, pay attention to your body and experiment to find what works for you.

When should you suspect ischemic colitis?

Ischemic colitis is a condition that can occur when blood flow to the colon becomes blocked. This can happen if the arteries that supply blood to the colon become narrowed or blocked. Ischemic colitis can also occur if the veins that drain blood away from the colon become blocked.

The most common symptom of ischemic colitis is abdominal pain. This pain is usually located in the lower left side of the abdomen. Other symptoms of ischemic colitis can include diarrhea, vomiting, and blood in the stool. Ischemic colitis can also cause fever, chills, and sweats.

If you experience any of these symptoms, you should see your doctor right away. Ischemic colitis is a serious condition that can lead to death if it is not treated promptly.

How common is Ischaemic colitis?

Ischaemic colitis (IC) is a medical condition that affects the large intestine and is a type of inflammatory bowel disease (IBD). IC is caused by a decrease in blood flow to the large intestine, which can happen as a result of a blockage in the arteries that supply blood to the intestine. This blockage can be caused by a clot or by a build-up of plaque in the arteries. IC is a relatively rare condition, and it is estimated that it affects between 1 and 4 in every 100,000 people.

The symptoms of IC vary depending on how much of the large intestine is affected by the decreased blood flow. In mild cases, the symptoms may be similar to those of other types of IBD, such as Crohn's disease or ulcerative colitis. These symptoms may include abdominal pain, bloating, and diarrhea. In more severe cases, the symptoms may include bloody stool, fever, and weight loss. In some cases, the decreased blood flow can lead to gangrene, which is the death of tissue due to a lack of blood flow.

IC is diagnosed through a combination of medical history, physical examination, and laboratory tests. The most common laboratory test used to diagnose IC is a colonoscopy. This test allows the doctor to look at the lining of the large intestine and look for signs of inflammation. The doctor may also take a biopsy, which is a small sample of tissue that is removed from the intestine and examined under a microscope.

There is no one specific treatment for IC. The goal of treatment is to improve the blood flow to the large intestine and to control the symptoms. Treatment may include medications, such as anti-inflammatory drugs, antibiotics, and pain relievers. In some cases, surgery may be necessary to remove the blockage from the arteries.

IC is a chronic condition, which means that it lasts for a long time. The symptoms may come and go, and they may be different from one person to the next. Some people may only have mild symptoms, while others may have more severe symptoms. With proper treatment, most people with IC are able to live normal, healthy lives.

Is yogurt good for ischemic colitis?

Ischemic colitis occurs when the blood supply to the colon becomes blocked. This can happen due to a variety of reasons, such as a narrowing of the arteries (arteriosclerosis) or a blood clot. When the blood supply is cut off, the tissue in the colon begins to die. This can lead to inflammation, pain, and diarrhea.

Yogurt has long been hailed as a health food, due to its high protein and calcium content, as well as its probiotic bacteria. Probiotics are live microorganisms that are believed to have health benefits when consumed. Some research has shown that probiotics may help to prevent or treat certain gastrointestinal disorders, such as inflammatory bowel disease (IBD) and infectious diarrhea.

It is not clear whether yogurt may help to treat ischemic colitis specifically. However, some studies have found that probiotic yogurt may help to reduce inflammation and improve symptoms in people with IBD. It is believed that the probiotic bacteria in yogurt may help to regulate the immune system and reduce inflammation in the gut.

If you are dealing with ischemic colitis, you should speak with your doctor before adding yogurt to your diet. yogurt may help to improve symptoms in some people, but it is not a cure for ischemic colitis. There is no one-size-fits-all approach to treating this condition, so it is important to work with your doctor to find the best treatment plan for you.

How do you treat ischemic colitis naturally?

There is no one-size-fits-all answer to this question, as the best way to treat ischemic colitis naturally will vary depending on the individual's unique situation and health condition. However, some general tips that may help include:

-Reducing stress levels: stress is a common trigger for ischemic colitis flare-ups, so finding ways to manage stress can be helpful in preventing and treating the condition.

-Eating a healthy diet: a diet rich in fiber, fruits, vegetables, and healthy fats can help to reduce inflammation and improve gut health.

-Exercising regularly: exercise has numerous health benefits, including reducing inflammation, improving gut health, and helping to manage stress levels.

-Taking probiotics: probiotics are live bacteria that are beneficial for gut health, and they may help to reduce the severity of ischemic colitis symptoms.

-Avoiding trigger foods: certain foods may trigger ischemic colitis symptoms, so it may be helpful to avoid these triggers. Common triggers include gluten, dairy, and spicy foods.

Is ischemic bowel painful?

Ischemic bowel, also known as mesenteric ischemia, is a condition in which not enough blood flow gets to the intestines. This can cause the intestines to become damaged and die. Ischemic bowel is a medical emergency, and it can be very painful.

The pain from ischemic bowel is usually severe and constant. It usually starts in the middle of the abdomen and radiates to the back. The pain may get worse when you move, take deep breaths, or lay down flat. You may also have other symptoms, such as nausea, vomiting, diarrhea, and constipation.

If you think you may have ischemic bowel, it's important to see a doctor right away. Ischemic bowel is a serious condition that can lead to death. Early diagnosis and treatment are important. Treatment for ischemic bowel may include medications, surgery, or a combination of both.

It is important to seek medical attention if you experience any symptoms of colitis, as it can be a potentially life-threatening condition. While there is no cure for colitis, there are treatments available that can help to manage the symptoms and improve the quality of life for those affected by the condition.

How does ischemia start?

Ischemia is a process whereby blood flow to a particular area is restricted. This can happen due to a number of reasons, including blockages in the arteries or veins, or damage to the blood vessels themselves. When ischemia occurs in the gut, it is known as colitis.

The exact mechanism by which ischemia starts is not fully understood, but it is thought to involve the narrowing of the blood vessels. This narrowing can be due to a build-up of plaque in the arteries, or to inflammation of the blood vessels. When the blood vessels are narrowed, they are unable to carry as much blood to the gut, and this can lead to tissue death.

Ischemia can also occur if there is a blockage in the veins that carry blood away from the gut. This blockage can be caused by a blood clot, or by damage to the veins. If blood flow is restricted in this way, it can again lead to tissue death.

Treatment for ischemia will depend on the underlying cause. If the cause is a blockage in the arteries, then treatment may involve surgery to remove the blockage. If the cause is a blockage in the veins, then treatment may involve using drugs to dissolve the blood clot. In some cases, surgery may be required to repair the damaged veins.

How do you get ischemic bowel?

There are a few different ways that ischemic bowel can develop. One way is when the blood supply to the bowel is blocked. This can happen if there is a blockage in the arteries that supply blood to the bowel. This blockage can be caused by a clot, a buildup of fatty deposits, or a narrowing of the arteries. Another way that ischemic bowel can develop is when the veins in the bowel are not working properly. This can cause the blood to pool in the veins and the blood supply to the bowel to be decreased. This can be caused by a blockage in the veins, a build-up of pressure in the veins, or a narrowing of the veins.

Does constipation cause ischemic colitis?

There are many different types of colitis, but ischemic colitis is one of the more severe forms. This condition is caused when there is not enough blood flow to the colon. This can be a problem because the colon needs blood to function properly.

There are many different things that can cause ischemic colitis. One of the more common causes is constipation. When someone is constipated, they are not able to have a regular bowel movement. This can cause the stool to become hard and dry. Hard stool can block the blood flow to the colon and cause ischemic colitis.

People who are constipated may also take laxatives to try to relieve their symptoms. However, laxatives can actually make ischemic colitis worse. This is because they can cause the colon to lose even more blood.

If you think you may be constipated, it is important to see a doctor. They can help you find the cause of your constipation and treat it. If you have ischemic colitis, it is important to get treatment right away. This condition can be very serious and even life-threatening.

Is ischemic colitis reversible?

Ischemic colitis is a condition that results when there is not enough blood flow to the colon. This can be due to a blockage in the arteries that supply blood to the colon, or it can be the result of a decrease in the amount of blood that is flowing to the area. When there is not enough blood flow, the cells of the colon begin to die, and this can lead to inflammation, bleeding, and other problems.

The good news is that ischemic colitis is often reversible. If the cause of the problem is a blockage in the arteries, then treatment can often be successful in opening up the arteries and restoring blood flow. If the cause is a decrease in blood flow, then treatment may be successful in increasing the amount of blood that is flowing to the area. In either case, the goal of treatment is to restore blood flow to the area and to reduce the inflammation and other problems that are associated with ischemic colitis.

Where does ischemic colitis most commonly occur?

Ischemic colitis is a medical condition that results when the blood flow to the colon is reduced. This can happen due to a number of different factors, but is most commonly seen in older adults. The reduced blood flow means that the colon doesn't get the oxygen and nutrients it needs, and this can cause the tissues to die. Ischemic colitis most commonly occurs in the elderly, and it is more common in men than in women. The exact cause of ischemic colitis is not known, but it is believed to be the result of a combination of factors. These include:

-Atherosclerosis: This is the narrowing of the arteries due to the buildup of plaque. This can reduce the blood flow to the colon and lead to ischemic colitis.

-Blood clots: These can form in the arteries and block the blood flow to the colon.

-Reduced blood pressure: This can happen due to various medical conditions, such as heart failure or septic shock.

-Reduced blood flow to the liver: This can happen due to cirrhosis or portal hypertension.

Ischemic colitis can also be caused by certain medications, such as non-steroidal anti-inflammatory drugs (NSAIDs) or chemotherapy drugs. In some cases, ischemic colitis may occur without any known cause.

How serious is ischemic bowel?

Ischemic bowel is a serious condition that can lead to death. It occurs when there is not enough blood flow to the intestines. This can happen if there is a blockage in the arteries that supply blood to the intestines. Ischemic bowel can also occur if there is a problem with the way the veins carry blood away from the intestines. If not treated, ischemic bowel can lead to death.

Can ischemic colitis be seen on CT scan?

Ischemic colitis is a condition that results when the blood supply to the colon is reduced. This can happen if the arteries that supply the blood to the colon are blocked or narrowed. When this happens, the cells in the colon can become damaged and die.

Ischemic colitis can be seen on a CT scan. The CT scan will show the areas of the colon where the blood supply is reduced. The CT scan will also show the areas of the colon where the cells are damaged.

Colitis is a debilitating and painful condition that can have a negative impact on a person's quality of life. While there is no cure for colitis, there are treatments available that can help to manage the symptoms and improve the person's quality of life.

What is the best drink for colitis?

There is no one-size-fits-all answer to this question, as the best drink for colitis may vary depending on the individual's symptoms and health status. However, some generally recommended drinks for people with colitis include water, clear soups, herbal teas, and diluted fruit juices. It is important to avoid caffeine, alcohol, and carbonated beverages, as these can worsen symptoms.

People with colitis may experience a range of symptoms, including abdominal pain, diarrhea, and blood in the stool. These symptoms can be debilitating and can lead to dehydration, so it is important to stay hydrated. Drinking plenty of fluids is crucial, and water is often the best choice. Clear soups and herbal teas can also help to keep the body hydrated and are easy on the stomach.

Fruit juices can be a good source of vitamins and minerals, but they should be diluted as they can be high in sugar. Avoiding caffeine, alcohol, and carbonated beverages is also important, as these can aggravate symptoms. Some people find that probiotic drinks, such as yogurt or kefir, help to reduce symptoms. Ultimately, it is important to work with a healthcare provider to determine the best diet for managing colitis.

What fruits are good for colitis?

A person with colitis may be wondering what fruits are good for their condition. While there are many opinions on which fruits are best, some general tips may be helpful. First, it is important to choose fruits that are easy to digest and low in fiber. Second, it is best to eat fruits that are fresh, as opposed to canned or processed. And lastly, it is important to eat a variety of fruits in order to get the most benefit.

Some specific fruits that are often recommended for people with colitis include bananas, papayas, and cantaloupe. These fruits are all low in fiber and easy to digest. They are also high in vitamins and minerals, which can be helpful for people with colitis. Other good choices include apricots, blueberries, and grapes. These fruits are also low in fiber and easy to digest, and they contain antioxidants, which can help to reduce inflammation.

Of course, every person is different and will tolerate different fruits differently. It is important to eat a variety of fruits and to pay attention to how your body reacts to them. If you find that a particular fruit bothers your stomach, you may want to avoid it or eat it in moderation. But in general, eating a diet that includes a variety of fresh fruits is a good idea for people with colitis.

Which is worse IBS or colitis?

There are two main types of inflammatory bowel diseases (IBD), ulcerative colitis (UC) and Crohn's disease (CD). Both diseases are chronic and can be debilitating, but they affect different parts of the digestive system. So, which is worse IBS or colitis?

To answer this question, we need to understand the difference between the two diseases. UC is a type of IBD that affects the large intestine, or colon. The lining of the colon becomes inflamed and ulcers may form. Crohn's disease, on the other hand, can affect any part of the digestive system from the mouth to the anus. The inflammation caused by Crohn's disease is often deeper, and can lead to the formation of fistulas (abnormal connections) between different organs.

While UC and Crohn's disease share many common symptoms, such as abdominal pain, cramping, diarrhea, fatigue, and weight loss, Crohn's disease is generally considered to be more severe. This is because Crohn's disease is more likely to lead to complications such as intestinal blockages, malnutrition, and even death. In contrast, UC is usually a lifelong condition, but it is not usually fatal.

So, to answer the question, which is worse IBS or colitis? Crohn's disease is generally considered to be more severe, but both diseases can be debilitating. If you have either UC or Crohn's disease, it is important to work with your doctor to develop a treatment plan that is right for you.

Is colitis a terminal illness?

No, colitis is not a terminal illness. It is a chronic condition that can lead to complications, such as intestinal bleeding and liver damage, but it is not fatal. While there is no cure for colitis, it can be managed with medication and lifestyle changes.

Is colitis brought on by stress?

Some experts believe that colitis may be brought on by stress, although more research is needed to confirm this. Stressful life events have been linked to the onset of colitis, and patients with colitis report higher levels of stress than those without the condition.

It is thought that stress may trigger an inflammatory response in the body that contributes to the development of colitis. Stressful life events may also disrupt the normal balance of bacteria in the gut, which is thought to play a role in the development of the condition.

If stress is a trigger for colitis, then managing stress may help to prevent flares. There are a number of stress-management techniques that may be helpful, including relaxation therapy, yoga, and meditation. Exercise and healthy eating habits can also help to reduce stress levels.

Can you live a long life with colitis?

There's no one-size-fits-all answer to this question, as the outlook for each person with colitis is different. Some people experience mild symptoms that come and go, while others have chronic, severe symptoms that can significantly reduce their life expectancy.

Factors that can affect the outlook for people with colitis include the type of colitis they have, how well their colitis is managed, and whether they develop any complications.

People with ulcerative colitis, for example, tend to have a better outlook than those with Crohn's disease. That's because ulcerative colitis is usually less likely to cause complications like fistulas (abnormal openings between organs) and intestinal strictures (narrowing of the intestine).

Those with Crohn's disease may also be more likely to develop other conditions like liver disease, arthritis, and skin problems.

People with colitis who smoke are also more likely to have more severe symptoms and a greater risk of complications. That's why quitting smoking is an important part of managing colitis.

Overall, the outlook for people with colitis has improved significantly in recent years. Thanks to advances in treatment, many people with colitis now enjoy long, healthy lives.

What vegetables should be avoided with colitis?

There are a few vegetables that should be avoided when you have colitis. These include:

- cabbage

- broccoli

- Brussel sprouts

- cauliflower

These vegetables contain a lot of insoluble fiber, which can aggravate the symptoms of colitis. They can also contribute to bloating and gas.

Other vegetables that you should eat in moderation if you have colitis include:

- Beans

- Corn

- Peas

- Onions

- garlic

These vegetables also contain insoluble fiber, but not as much as the vegetables that should be avoided. They may still aggravate your symptoms, but they are not as likely to do so.

If you have colitis, you should also avoid eating spicy foods. Spicy foods can irritate the lining of your intestine, which can make your symptoms worse.

While there is no cure for colitis, it is possible to manage the condition with medication and lifestyle changes. In some cases, surgery may be necessary to remove the diseased portion of the intestine. With proper treatment, people with colitis can lead normal, healthy lives.

Is colitis a side effect of radiation?

While colitis may occur as a result of radiation therapy, this does not mean that it is a side effect of the treatment. Colitis is a condition of the large intestine, characterized by inflammation and ulceration of the inner lining of the colon. The most common symptom of colitis is abdominal pain, often accompanied by diarrhea.

There are many possible causes of colitis, including infections, inflammatory bowel diseases, and autoimmune disorders. Radiation therapy can also cause inflammation of the colon, but this is typically not considered to be a side effect of the treatment.

Radiation therapy is a common treatment for cancer, and it can be an effective way to kill cancer cells. However, radiation therapy can also damage healthy cells, leading to side effects. The side effects of radiation therapy depend on the type and dose of radiation used, as well as the part of the body that is being treated.

Common side effects of radiation therapy include fatigue, skin reactions, and diarrhea. These side effects are usually temporary and go away after treatment is completed. However, radiation therapy can also cause long-term side effects, such as colitis.

Colitis is a condition that can be caused by radiation therapy, but it is not a side effect of the treatment. Colitis is a condition of the large intestine, characterized by inflammation and ulceration of the inner lining of the colon. The most common symptom of colitis is abdominal pain, often accompanied by diarrhea.

There are many possible causes of colitis, including infections, inflammatory bowel diseases, and autoimmune disorders. Radiation therapy can also cause inflammation of the colon, but this is typically not considered to be a side effect of the treatment.

To date, there is no definitive evidence that radiation therapy causes colitis. However, if you develop colitis after radiation therapy, it is important to see a doctor so that the condition can be properly diagnosed and treated.

What is the cure for radiation proctitis?

Radiation proctitis is a type of proctitis, which is an inflammation of the rectum. The most common symptom of radiation proctitis is bleeding from the rectum. Other symptoms include diarrhea, abdominal pain, and tenesmus (rectal pain that is relieved by passing stool).

There is no cure for radiation proctitis, but there are treatment options that can help relieve symptoms. The most common treatment is steroids, which can be taken orally or rectally. Steroids help to reduce inflammation and bleeding. Other treatments include anti-inflammatory medications, such as 5-aminosalicylates, and surgery.

5-aminosalicylates are a type of medication that is commonly used to treat inflammatory bowel diseases, such as Crohn's disease and ulcerative colitis. 5-aminosalicylates work by reducing inflammation in the intestines. The most common 5-aminosalicylate is mesalamine, which is available in many different forms, including enemas, suppositories, and pills.

Surgery is an option for people who have severe symptoms that do not respond to other treatments. Surgery is usually only considered if other treatments have failed. The most common type of surgery for radiation proctitis is a colostomy, which is when the end of the large intestine is brought through an opening in the abdominal wall. This allows stool to pass into a bag, which is then emptied when necessary.

Does radiation proctitis ever heal?

Radiation proctitis is a side effect of radiation therapy that can cause inflammation and ulceration in the lining of the rectum. Although the symptoms of radiation proctitis can be debilitating, the good news is that the condition is usually reversible and often goes away on its own within a few months to a year after treatment. In some cases, however, radiation proctitis may be more persistent, and require medical treatment.

If you are receiving radiation therapy for cancer, it is important to be aware of the possible side effects, including radiation proctitis. This condition is caused by exposure to high-energy radiation, which damages the lining of the rectum. Symptoms of radiation proctitis can include rectal bleeding, diarrhea, urgency to have a bowel movement, and cramping. In some cases, radiation proctitis can also lead to rectal pain, urinary frequency, and incontinence.

Although the symptoms of radiation proctitis can be unpleasant, the condition is usually reversible. In most cases, the symptoms improve within a few months to a year after treatment. In some cases, however, radiation proctitis may be more persistent, and require medical treatment.

If you are experiencing symptoms of radiation proctitis, it is important to see your doctor. Your doctor can perform a physical exam and order tests to confirm the diagnosis. Once the diagnosis is confirmed, your doctor will work with you to develop a treatment plan.

In most cases, the symptoms of radiation proctitis can be managed with lifestyle changes and over-the-counter medications. If your symptoms are more severe, you may require prescription medication or surgery.

Radiation proctitis is a serious condition, but it is important to remember that it is usually reversible. With early diagnosis and proper treatment, most people with radiation proctitis can recover and return to their normal activities.

How long does radiation colitis last?

Radiation colitis is a type of inflammation of the colon that can occur after radiation therapy to the abdomen. The symptoms of radiation colitis include abdominal pain, bloody diarrhea, and weight loss. Most cases of radiation colitis resolve within a few months, but some cases can last for years.

Radiation colitis is more likely to occur in people who have had a previous history of inflammatory bowel disease, such as Crohn's disease or ulcerative colitis. People who have received radiation therapy for cancer are also at risk for developing radiation colitis.

Treatment for radiation colitis includes anti-inflammatory medications, such as steroids, and antidiarrheal medications. In severe cases, surgery may be necessary to remove part of the inflamed colon.

People who have received radiation therapy should be sure to follow up with their doctor and report any new or worsening symptoms.

How do you get radiation colitis?

Radiation colitis is a type of bowel inflammation that can occur after having radiation therapy. The large intestine and rectum are exposed to high doses of radiation during this treatment, which can damage the lining of these organs and lead to inflammation. Symptoms of radiation colitis include diarrhea, abdominal pain, and rectal bleeding. This condition can be very serious, and it is important to see a doctor if you experience any of these symptoms.

There are a few different ways that radiation colitis can develop. One is when the healthy cells in the lining of the intestine are damaged by the radiation therapy. This damage can lead to inflammation and can cause the symptoms listed above. Another way that radiation colitis can develop is when the blood vessels in the intestine are damaged by the radiation therapy. This can cause bleeding and can also lead to inflammation.

Radiation colitis is a serious condition that can be very painful and debilitating. If you are experiencing any of the symptoms listed above, it is important to see a doctor as soon as possible. There are treatments available that can help to ease the symptoms of this condition and help you to feel better.

What organ is affected by colitis?

The organ most affected by colitis is the large intestine, also known as the colon. The colon is a long, coiled tube that removes water and salt from solid waste before it leaves the body. Colitis is an inflammation of the colon that can cause a variety of symptoms, including abdominal pain, diarrhea, and bloating. The exact cause of colitis is unknown, but it is believed to be a combination of genetic and environmental factors.

What are the 2 most common side effects of radiation?

Radiation therapy is a common treatment for cancer, but it can also come with some side effects. The two most common side effects of radiation are fatigue and skin reactions. Fatigue can be caused by the treatment itself or from the anxiety and stress of dealing with a cancer diagnosis. Skin reactions are also common, as the radiation can cause the skin to become dry, red, and irritated. These side effects can be bothersome, but they usually go away after the treatment is over.

In conclusion, colitis is a debilitating and painful condition that can have a serious impact on a person's quality of life. While there is no cure for colitis, there are treatments available that can help to manage the symptoms and improve the person's quality of life. With the right medical care and support, people with colitis can often lead relatively normal lives.

How is radiation induced colitis treated?

Radiation induced colitis is a type of colitis that is caused by exposure to radiation. There are two types of radiation therapy: external radiation therapy and internal radiation therapy. External radiation therapy uses a machine outside of the body to target the cancer. Internal radiation therapy uses a device called a brachytherapy, which is placed inside the body near the cancer.

Radiation induced colitis can be a side effect of radiation therapy. The severity of the colitis depends on the dose of radiation and the area of the body that is being treated. The most common symptom of radiation induced colitis is diarrhea. Other symptoms may include rectal bleeding, abdominal pain, and cramping.

Radiation therapy is the main treatment for radiation induced colitis. The goal of radiation therapy is to lower the dose of radiation to the surrounding healthy tissue. This can be done by reducing the number of treatments, changing the type of radiation, or lowering the dose of radiation.

Some other treatments for radiation induced colitis may include:

-Anti-diarrheal medications: These medications can help to control the diarrhea.

-Pain medications: These medications can help to control the pain and cramping.

-Steroids: These medications can help to decrease inflammation.

-Surgery: In some cases, surgery may be necessary to remove the damaged intestine.

What happens if proctitis is left untreated?

If proctitis is left untreated, the inflammation may spread to the large intestine, a condition known as colitis. This can lead to a number of serious complications, including bleeding, ulceration, and even perforation of the intestine. In severe cases, colitis can be fatal. Early diagnosis and treatment of proctitis is therefore essential to preventing these potentially life-threatening complications.

What is the difference between colitis and proctitis?

Colitis and proctitis are both medical conditions that involve inflammation of the intestine. However, there are some key differences between the two conditions.

Proctitis is an inflammation of the rectum, which is the final portion of the large intestine. This condition can be caused by a variety of factors, including infection, allergies, and autoimmune disorders. Symptoms of proctitis may include rectal bleeding, pain, and diarrhea.

Colitis, on the other hand, is an inflammation of the large intestine (colon). This condition can also be caused by a variety of factors, including infection, allergies, and autoimmune disorders. However, colitis is often associated with inflammatory bowel diseases (IBD), such as Crohn's disease and ulcerative colitis. Symptoms of colitis may include abdominal pain, bloody stool, and weight loss.

While both colitis and proctitis can be painful and disruptive, colitis is generally considered to be a more serious condition. This is because colitis can lead to IBD, which can be a chronic and debilitating condition. If you think you may be suffering from either condition, it is important to see a doctor for a diagnosis.

Is radiation proctitis serious?

Radiation proctitis is a rare but serious complication that can occur after radiation therapy to the pelvis. The condition results in inflammation of the rectum and can cause a variety of symptoms, including bleeding, pain, and difficulty with bowel movements. In some cases, radiation proctitis can lead to more serious problems, such as fistulas (abnormal connections between different parts of the body) or colorectal cancer.

Although radiation proctitis is a serious condition, it is important to remember that it is rare. The vast majority of people who undergo radiation therapy will not develop this complication. If you do develop radiation proctitis, it is important to see a doctor so that the condition can be treated. With prompt and proper treatment, most people with radiation proctitis can manage their symptoms and live normal, healthy lives.

Is Metamucil good for radiation proctitis?

Radiation proctitis is a condition that can be caused by radiation therapy to the pelvis. The radiotherapy can damage the lining of the rectum, which can lead to inflammation and bleeding. Metamucil is a fiber supplement that is sometimes used to treat constipation. It is not clear if Metamucil is effective for radiation proctitis. Some studies suggest that it may help to reduce symptoms, but more research is needed. If you are considering using Metamucil for radiation proctitis, talk to your doctor first to see if it is right for you.

Is proctitis hard to treat?

Proctitis is a medical condition that affects the rectum and anal area. The main symptom of proctitis is rectal pain. This pain can be severe and can make it difficult to have a bowel movement. Other symptoms of proctitis include rectal bleeding, diarrhea, and constipation.

Proctitis is usually caused by an infection, but it can also be caused by other medical conditions such as Crohn's disease, irritable bowel syndrome, or cancer. Treatment for proctitis depends on the cause. Infections are typically treated with antibiotics. Other medical conditions may require different treatments.

Proctitis can be a difficult condition to treat. The main symptom, rectal pain, can be severe and difficult to manage. If the proctitis is caused by an infection, it is important to finish the full course of antibiotics to ensure the infection is completely gone. Other medical conditions that can cause proctitis may require more long-term treatment.

Despite the challenges of treating proctitis, many people are able to effectively manage their condition and live relatively normal lives.

Does colitis shorten lifespan?

Although the answer to this question may seem simple, the truth is that colitis does not technically shorten lifespan. However, the chronic inflammation of the colon associated with colitis can lead to serious health complications, which may reduce life expectancy.

left untreated, colitis can cause a number of potentially life-threatening complications, such as liver disease, cancer, and sepsis (blood poisoning). While there is no cure for colitis, prompt and effective treatment can help to control the symptoms and prevent these serious complications from developing.

With proper treatment, most people with colitis are able to enjoy a normal lifespan. However, it is important to be aware of the potential risks and to seek medical help as soon as possible if you experience any symptoms of colitis.

There are many different types of colitis, each with its own set of symptoms and treatment options. Some forms of colitis can be mild, while others can be quite severe. Regardless of the type of colitis you have, it is important to see a doctor if you are experiencing any symptoms. With proper treatment, most people with colitis can live normal, healthy lives.

Why does colitis start?

Inflammatory bowel diseases like colitis usually start when the body's immune system mistakenly attacks the intestines. Doctors don't know exactly why this happens, but it may be triggered by a virus or bacteria. Other possible causes include:

- genes

- smoking

- a diet high in animal fat

- a history of other autoimmune diseases

The exact cause of colitis is still unknown, but researchers have identified several possible risk factors. It is thought that a combination of genetic and environmental factors may play a role in the development of the disease.

What does colitis turn into?

When referring to colitis, many people are wondering what the long-term effects may be. In some cases, colitis may go away on its own after a few weeks. However, there are also instances where the colitis may become a chronic condition. When this happens, the inflammation does not go away and may even cause the intestines to become damaged. This damage can lead to various complications, some of which can be life-threatening.

One serious complication that can result from colitis is malnutrition. This is because the inflammation can cause the intestines to absorb nutrients less effectively. Additionally, people with chronic colitis may also have nausea and vomiting, which can lead to further nutrient loss. Without proper nutrition, the body will not be able to function properly and may even begin to break down muscle tissue for energy.

Another complication that can occur as a result of colitis is intestinal blockage. This happens when the inflammation causes the intestines to swell and narrow. This can cause food or waste to get stuck, leading to pain and vomiting. In severe cases, the blockage can cut off blood flow to the intestines and may even require surgery to correct.

Lastly, colitis can also lead to an increased risk of developing colon cancer. This is because the inflammation can cause DNA damage to the cells lining the colon. This damage can lead to the development of precancerous growths, which may eventually turn into cancer. While the risk of developing colon cancer is still relatively low, it is important to be aware of the potential complication.

If you are experiencing any symptoms of colitis, it is important to see a doctor for a proper diagnosis. While colitis is not typically a serious condition, the potential complications can be severe. With early diagnosis and treatment, the majority of people with colitis will be able to live relatively normal, healthy lives.

What is the best medication for colitis?

There are many different medications that can be used to treat colitis, and the best medication for each individual may vary depending on the severity of their symptoms. Some common medications that are used to treat colitis include anti-inflammatory drugs, antibiotics, and immunosuppressive agents. In mild cases of colitis, over-the-counter anti-inflammatory medications such as ibuprofen may be sufficient to relieve symptoms. More severe cases may require prescription medications such as corticosteroids or immunosuppressive agents. In some cases, surgery may be necessary to remove the diseased portion of the colon.

What is the difference between colitis and colitis?

The terms colitis and Crohn's disease are often used interchangeably, but there are distinct differences between the two. Colitis is a chronic inflammation of the large intestine, also known as the colon. Crohn's disease is a chronic inflammation of the entire gastrointestinal tract, from the mouth to the anus. The main difference between the two is the location of the inflammation.

Colitis is caused by a variety of things, including infection, autoimmune disease, and allergies. Crohn's disease is thought to be caused by a combination of environmental, genetic, and immunological factors. The exact cause is unknown.

Colitis can be treated with a number of different medications, including anti-inflammatories, antibiotics, and immune suppressants. Crohn's disease is more difficult to treat, and often requires a combination of medication and surgery.

If you think you may have either colitis or Crohn's disease, it is important to see a doctor for a diagnosis. These conditions can both be extremely uncomfortable and can lead to serious complications if left untreated.

Which organ is most affected by radiation?

Besides cancer, another serious health concern associated with radiation is its effect on the digestive system, specifically the colon. The organ that is most affected by radiation is the large intestine, or colon. The mucous membranes that line the inside of the colon are very sensitive to radiation and can be easily damaged. This can lead to a number of serious health problems, including bleeding, infection, and inflammation.

Radiation therapy is a common treatment for cancer, and it works by damaging the DNA of cancer cells. This makes it difficult for them to grow and multiply. However, radiation therapy can also damage the DNA of healthy cells, including the cells that line the colon. This can cause a number of side effects, including diarrhea, constipation, and abdominal pain. In some cases, radiation therapy can also lead to more serious problems, such as colitis.

Colitis is a condition that causes inflammation of the lining of the colon. This can lead to a number of symptoms, including diarrhea, abdominal pain, and bleeding. Colitis is a serious condition that can be life-threatening. If you are undergoing radiation therapy, it is important to be aware of the potential risks and talk to your doctor about how to minimize them.

What are the major permanent side effects of radiation?

Radiation therapy is a common treatment for cancer, and it can be very effective in killing cancer cells. However, like all treatments, it comes with some risks and side effects. While most side effects are temporary and will go away after treatment is complete, there are some that can be long-lasting or even permanent.

One of the most common long-term side effects of radiation therapy is fatigue. You may feel tired all the time and have less energy than usual. This can last for weeks or even months after treatment. Radiation can also cause skin changes. The skin in the treatment area may become dry, red, and irritated. It may also become more sensitive to the sun. These changes usually go away after treatment, but in some cases, they can be permanent.

Radiation therapy can also damage the tissues and organs in the treatment area. This can lead to long-term problems such as digestive issues, urinary problems, and infertility. In some cases, these problems can be very serious and even life-threatening.

If you are receiving radiation therapy, it is important to talk to your doctor about the potential risks and side effects. They can help you understand what to expect and how to manage any long-term effects.

What part of the body is most affected by radiation?

Radiation therapy affects the entire body, but the tissues and organs that are most sensitive to radiation are those that divide the fastest. This includes the cells lining the gastrointestinal tract, as well as the bone marrow, which produces blood cells. Radiation can also damage the heart, lungs, and central nervous system.

There is no one answer to the question of how to treat colitis. Some people find that their symptoms improve with lifestyle changes like eating a healthy diet, reducing stress, and getting regular exercise. Others may need medication or surgery to get their symptoms under control. If you have colitis, it's important to work with your doctor to find a treatment plan that's right for you.

When does radiation enteritis start?

Radiation enteritis usually starts within a few days of beginning radiation therapy, though it may take up to a couple of weeks for symptoms to develop. The most common symptom is diarrhoea, which may be mild to severe. Other symptoms may include abdominal pain, cramping, bloating, gas, nausea, and vomiting. The intensity of symptoms varies from person to person and can depend on the type and dose of radiation therapy being received. Usually, symptoms improve once radiation therapy is finished. In some cases, however, radiation enteritis may be a long-term condition.

What is the best natural remedy for radiation proctitis?

Radiation therapy is a common treatment for cancer that can sometimes lead to proctitis, or inflammation of the rectum.

There are a number of natural remedies that may help to reduce the symptoms of radiation proctitis. These include dietary changes, herbal supplements, and home remedies.

Dietary changes that may help to reduce inflammation include avoiding trigger foods, eating more anti-inflammatory foods, and increasing fiber intake. Herbal supplements that may help to reduce inflammation include turmeric, ginger, and boswellia. Home remedies that may help to reduce inflammation include hot sitz baths, cold compress, and aloe vera.

radiation proctitis can be a difficult condition to manage, but there are a number of natural remedies that may help to reduce symptoms. It is important to work with a healthcare professional to find the best treatment plan for you.

How do you calm colitis?

When you have colitis, the last thing you want to do is eat. You may not feel like eating because of the stomach pain or because you are worried about going to the bathroom. However, not eating can make your colitis worse. You need to eat to give your body the energy it needs to heal.

There are a few things you can do to make eating easier when you have colitis. First, eat small meals throughout the day instead of three large meals. It may be easier on your stomach to eat several small meals than to eat a large meal and then have to wait a long time for your next meal.

Second, eat slowly. It can be tempting to gulp your food down when you are hungry, but eating too fast can make your colitis worse. Eating slowly will help you eat less and will give your body time to digest your food properly.

Third, avoid foods that are hard to digest. Foods that are high in fiber can be hard on your stomach when you have colitis. You may want to avoid eating raw vegetables, whole grains, and nuts. Instead, eat cooked vegetables, white rice, and peeled fruits.

Fourth, avoid trigger foods. Everybody is different, so you will need to figure out which foods make your colitis worse. Some common trigger foods include dairy, caffeine, alcohol, and spicy foods. If you eat a food that triggers your colitis, you may want to eat smaller amounts of that food or avoid it altogether.

Finally, stay hydrated. Drinking enough water is important for everybody, but it is especially important when you have colitis. Drinking water will help to soften your stool and will make it easier to go to the bathroom. You may also want to drink other clear fluids, such as broth or juice.

How long does it take to recover from a colitis flare-up?

When talking about how long it takes to recover from a colitis flare up, it is important to keep in mind that there is no one definitive answer. The length of time it takes to recover can vary greatly from person to person, and even from flare-up to flare-up.

There are a few factors that can affect how long it takes to recover from a colitis flare-up. The first is the severity of the flare-up. A milder flare-up will obviously take less time to recover from than a more severe one. The second factor is how well you manage the flare-up. If you take care of yourself and get plenty of rest, you will recover more quickly than if you do not. The third factor is how your body responds to treatment. Some people respond very well to medication and other treatments and recover quickly, while others do not.

All of that being said, in general, it takes most people a week or two to recover from a colitis flare-up. However, some people may take longer, and some people may have shorter recoveries. The best thing you can do is to listen to your body and give yourself the time you need to recover.

How do you stop colitis symptoms?

If you're experiencing symptoms of colitis, it's important to seek medical attention. Once you've been diagnosed, your doctor will work with you to develop a treatment plan. There are a number of different ways to treat colitis, and the best approach depends on the severity of your symptoms and the underlying cause of your condition.

In general, the goal of treatment is to reduce inflammation and help your digestive system heal. Depending on the severity of your symptoms, this may be accomplished with medication, changes to your diet, or both.

Medications typically used to treat colitis include anti-inflammatory drugs, immune-suppressing drugs, and antibiotics. These medications can help reduce inflammation, improve symptoms, and prevent complications.

In some cases, dietary changes may also be recommended. For example, if you have ulcerative colitis, you may be advised to avoid triggering foods, such as spicy foods or dairy products. A dietitian can provide guidance on how to modify your diet to help manage your symptoms.

The specific treatment approach depends on the underlying cause of your colitis. Treatment may be more aggressive for Crohn's disease, for example, while ulcerative colitis is often treated with a more conservative approach.

No matter what type of colitis you have, it's important to work with your doctor to develop a treatment plan that's right for you. With treatment, most people are able to effectively manage their symptoms and enjoy a good quality of life.

There is no one-size-fits-all approach to managing colitis, as the condition can vary significantly from person to person. However, there are some basic steps that everyone with colitis can take to help manage the condition and reduce the risk of flares. These include staying hydrated, eating a nutritious diet, getting regular exercise, and avoiding stress. If you have severe colitis, you may also need to take medication to keep the condition under control. With proper management, many people with colitis are able to lead normal, active lives.

SD - #0040 - 140926 - C0 - 229/152/12 - PB - 9781776969760 - Matt Lamination